OF NIGHTMARES AND MIRACLES
A COVID-19 SURVIVAL STORY

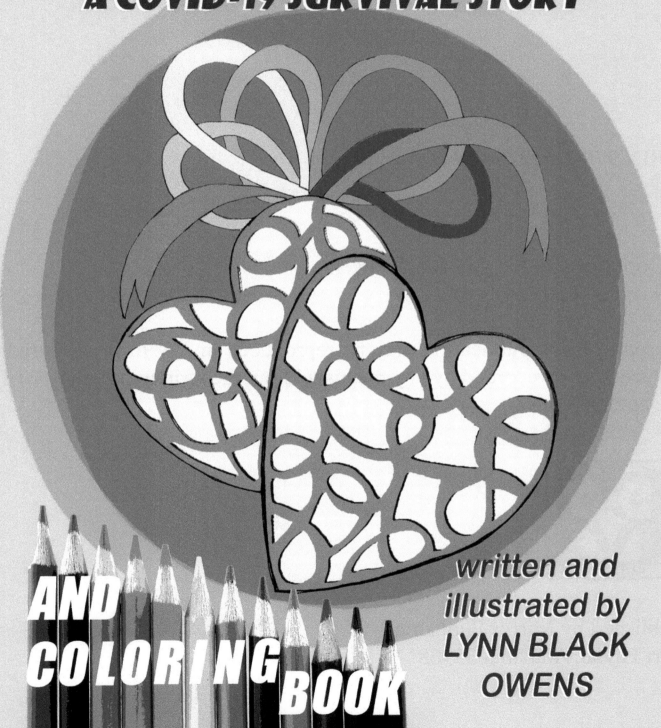

written and
illustrated by
LYNN BLACK
OWENS

AND COLORING BOOK

ISBN 978-1-61225-473-9

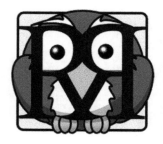

Published by Mirror Publishing
Fort Payne, Alabama 35968

Printed in the USA.

I would like to dedicate this book to my dad. And to all the healthcare workers at all three facilities. And to my pastor, Kent Wilborn, who visited me every chance he got and who fought his own miracle battle with COVID-19. And to my family, my church family, and my friends who prayed for me.

A Special Note from the Author

There was this young man who wasn't a doctor or nurse; he worked in housekeeping. He had been coming in my room to clean the entire time I was in ICU at Gadsden Regional. The first day I was awake enough to notice people, he came in to clean. He was so surprised to see me awake. When he came in, he happily told me how thankful he was that I was awake, that he had been watching me and praying for me. He said I had scared him because I was so bad and had been on the ventilator so long. Each day he came in, he was a joy to be around. I wish everyone, no matter what position you hold, would do their job like he does. Even though my doctors and nurses will always be remembered, I will always remember Anthony. We should hope that people remember us for doing a good job and being kind no matter what we do.

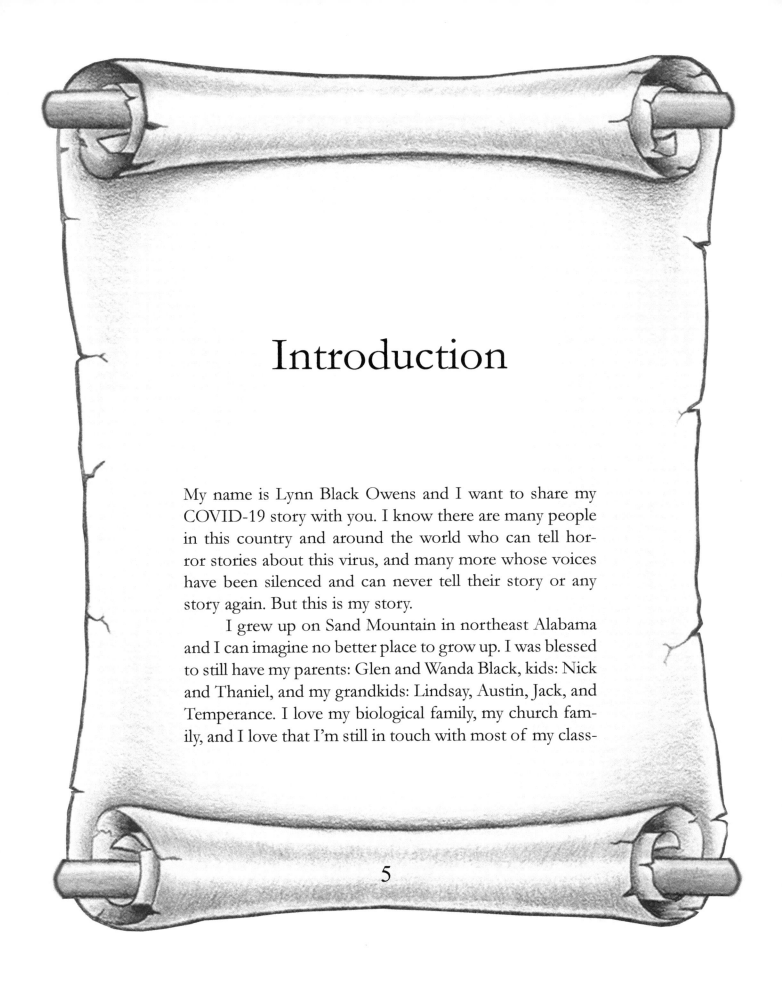

Introduction

My name is Lynn Black Owens and I want to share my COVID-19 story with you. I know there are many people in this country and around the world who can tell horror stories about this virus, and many more whose voices have been silenced and can never tell their story or any story again. But this is my story.

I grew up on Sand Mountain in northeast Alabama and I can imagine no better place to grow up. I was blessed to still have my parents: Glen and Wanda Black, kids: Nick and Thaniel, and my grandkids: Lindsay, Austin, Jack, and Temperance. I love my biological family, my church family, and I love that I'm still in touch with most of my class-

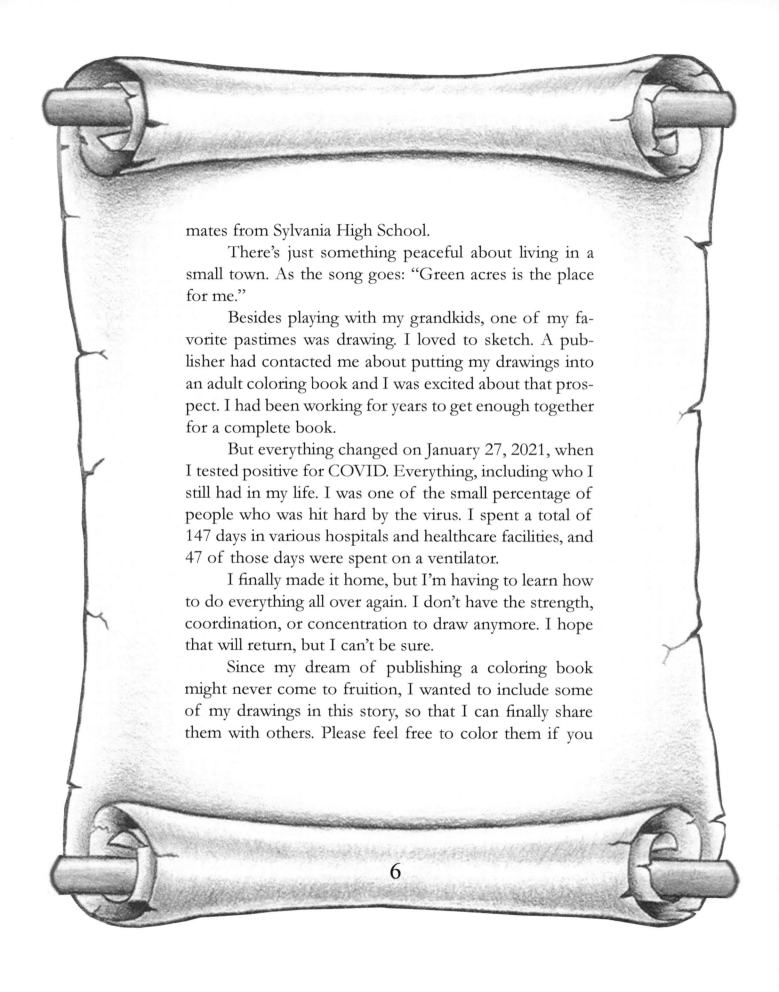

mates from Sylvania High School.

There's just something peaceful about living in a small town. As the song goes: "Green acres is the place for me."

Besides playing with my grandkids, one of my favorite pastimes was drawing. I loved to sketch. A publisher had contacted me about putting my drawings into an adult coloring book and I was excited about that prospect. I had been working for years to get enough together for a complete book.

But everything changed on January 27, 2021, when I tested positive for COVID. Everything, including who I still had in my life. I was one of the small percentage of people who was hit hard by the virus. I spent a total of 147 days in various hospitals and healthcare facilities, and 47 of those days were spent on a ventilator.

I finally made it home, but I'm having to learn how to do everything all over again. I don't have the strength, coordination, or concentration to draw anymore. I hope that will return, but I can't be sure.

Since my dream of publishing a coloring book might never come to fruition, I wanted to include some of my drawings in this story, so that I can finally share them with others. Please feel free to color them if you

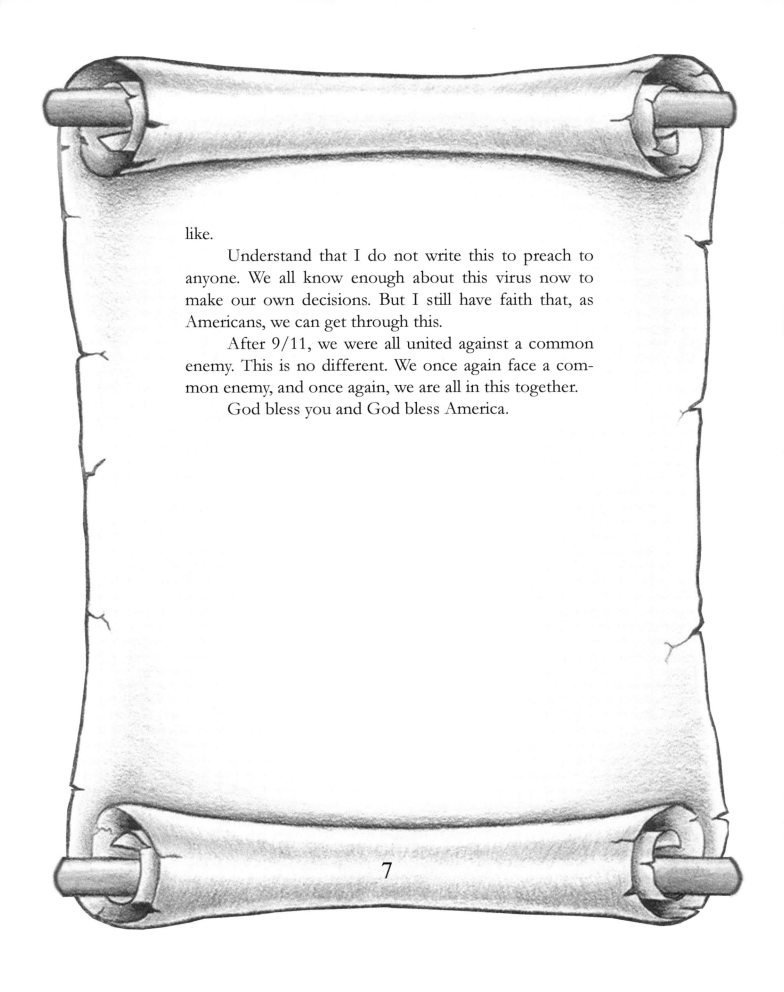

like.

Understand that I do not write this to preach to anyone. We all know enough about this virus now to make our own decisions. But I still have faith that, as Americans, we can get through this.

After 9/11, we were all united against a common enemy. This is no different. We once again face a common enemy, and once again, we are all in this together.

God bless you and God bless America.

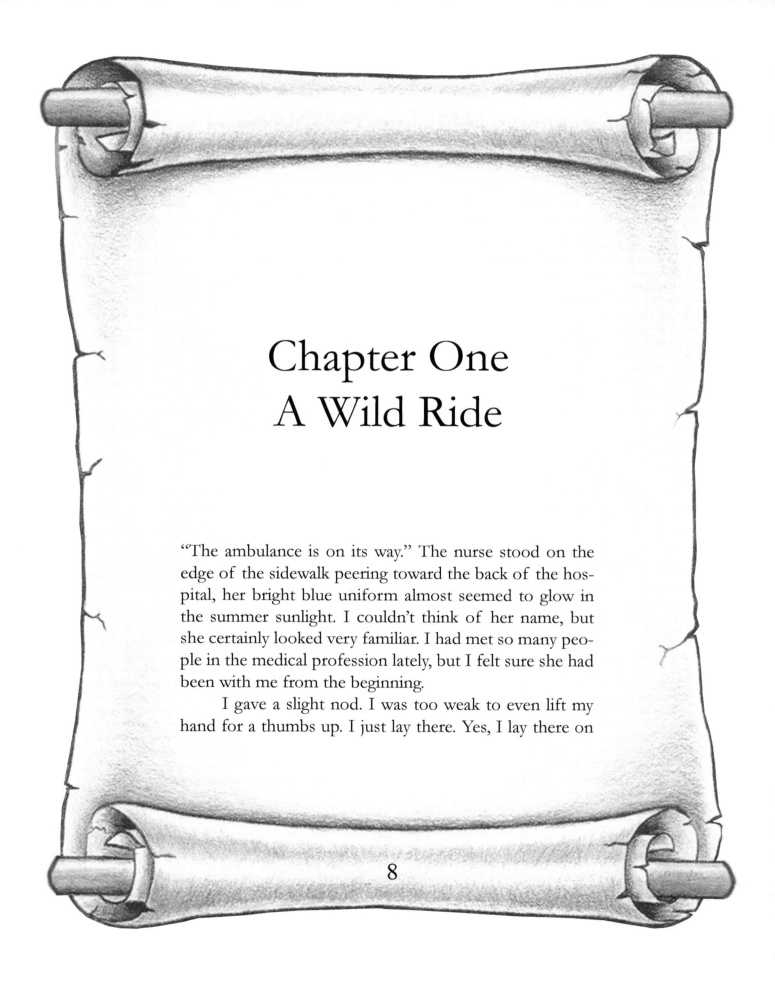

Chapter One
A Wild Ride

"The ambulance is on its way." The nurse stood on the edge of the sidewalk peering toward the back of the hospital, her bright blue uniform almost seemed to glow in the summer sunlight. I couldn't think of her name, but she certainly looked very familiar. I had met so many people in the medical profession lately, but I felt sure she had been with me from the beginning.

I gave a slight nod. I was too weak to even lift my hand for a thumbs up. I just lay there. Yes, I lay there on

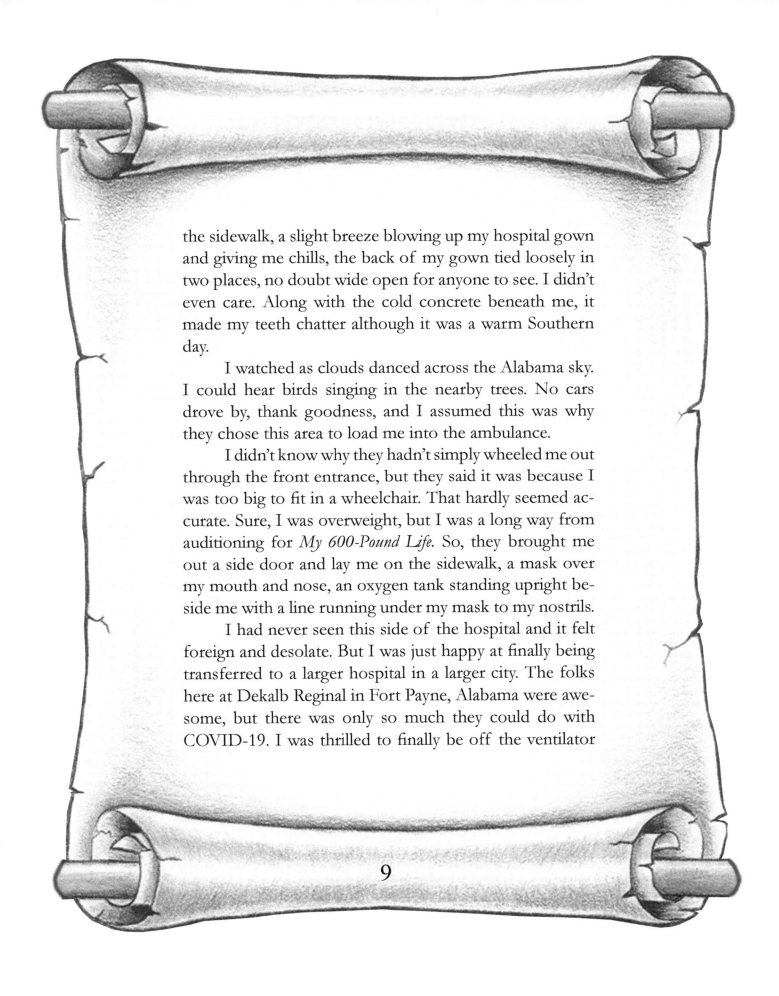

the sidewalk, a slight breeze blowing up my hospital gown and giving me chills, the back of my gown tied loosely in two places, no doubt wide open for anyone to see. I didn't even care. Along with the cold concrete beneath me, it made my teeth chatter although it was a warm Southern day.

I watched as clouds danced across the Alabama sky. I could hear birds singing in the nearby trees. No cars drove by, thank goodness, and I assumed this was why they chose this area to load me into the ambulance.

I didn't know why they hadn't simply wheeled me out through the front entrance, but they said it was because I was too big to fit in a wheelchair. That hardly seemed accurate. Sure, I was overweight, but I was a long way from auditioning for *My 600-Pound Life*. So, they brought me out a side door and lay me on the sidewalk, a mask over my mouth and nose, an oxygen tank standing upright beside me with a line running under my mask to my nostrils.

I had never seen this side of the hospital and it felt foreign and desolate. But I was just happy at finally being transferred to a larger hospital in a larger city. The folks here at Dekalb Reginal in Fort Payne, Alabama were awesome, but there was only so much they could do with COVID-19. I was thrilled to finally be off the ventilator

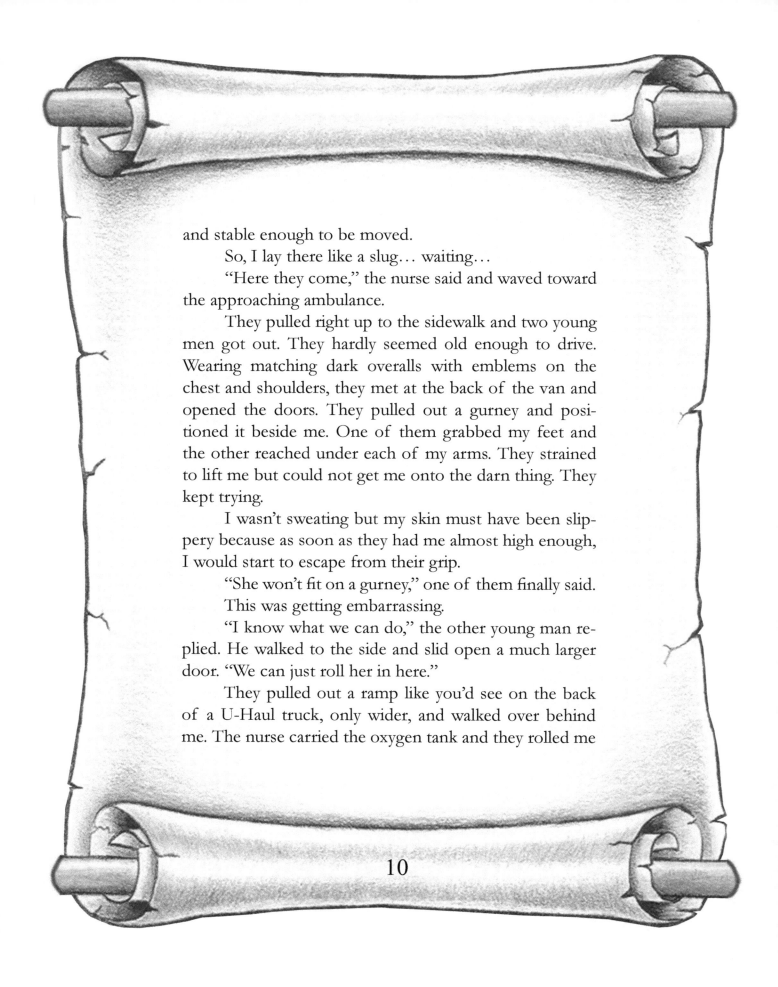

and stable enough to be moved.

So, I lay there like a slug… waiting…

"Here they come," the nurse said and waved toward the approaching ambulance.

They pulled right up to the sidewalk and two young men got out. They hardly seemed old enough to drive. Wearing matching dark overalls with emblems on the chest and shoulders, they met at the back of the van and opened the doors. They pulled out a gurney and positioned it beside me. One of them grabbed my feet and the other reached under each of my arms. They strained to lift me but could not get me onto the darn thing. They kept trying.

I wasn't sweating but my skin must have been slippery because as soon as they had me almost high enough, I would start to escape from their grip.

"She won't fit on a gurney," one of them finally said.

This was getting embarrassing.

"I know what we can do," the other young man replied. He walked to the side and slid open a much larger door. "We can just roll her in here."

They pulled out a ramp like you'd see on the back of a U-Haul truck, only wider, and walked over behind me. The nurse carried the oxygen tank and they rolled me

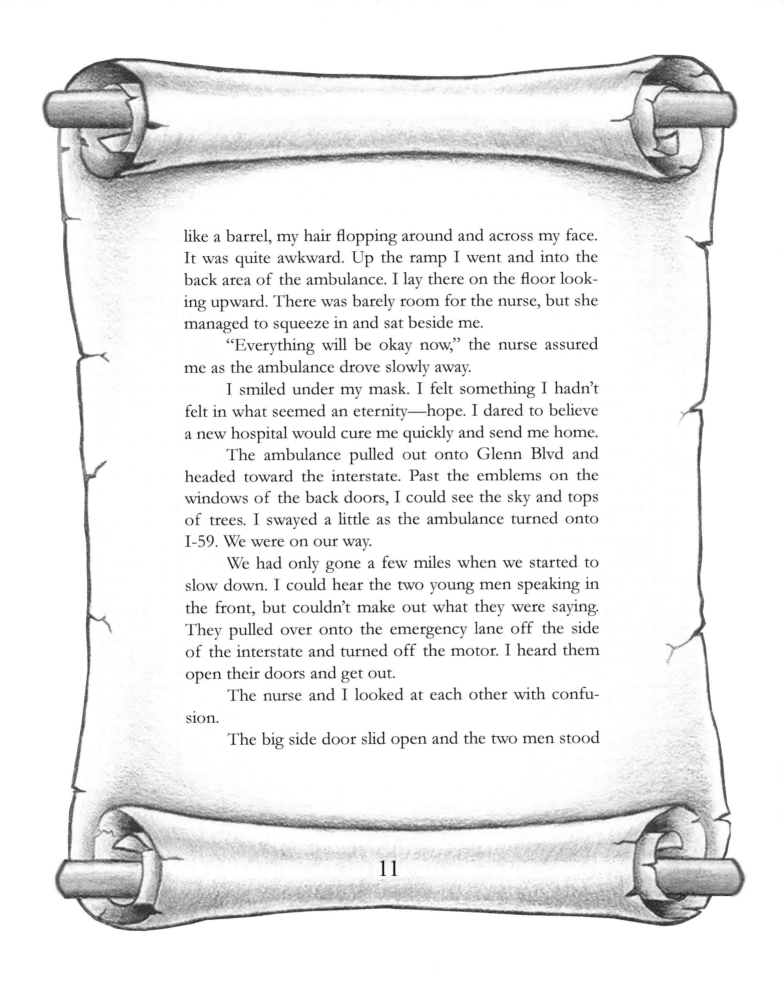

like a barrel, my hair flopping around and across my face. It was quite awkward. Up the ramp I went and into the back area of the ambulance. I lay there on the floor looking upward. There was barely room for the nurse, but she managed to squeeze in and sat beside me.

"Everything will be okay now," the nurse assured me as the ambulance drove slowly away.

I smiled under my mask. I felt something I hadn't felt in what seemed an eternity—hope. I dared to believe a new hospital would cure me quickly and send me home.

The ambulance pulled out onto Glenn Blvd and headed toward the interstate. Past the emblems on the windows of the back doors, I could see the sky and tops of trees. I swayed a little as the ambulance turned onto I-59. We were on our way.

We had only gone a few miles when we started to slow down. I could hear the two young men speaking in the front, but couldn't make out what they were saying. They pulled over onto the emergency lane off the side of the interstate and turned off the motor. I heard them open their doors and get out.

The nurse and I looked at each other with confusion.

The big side door slid open and the two men stood

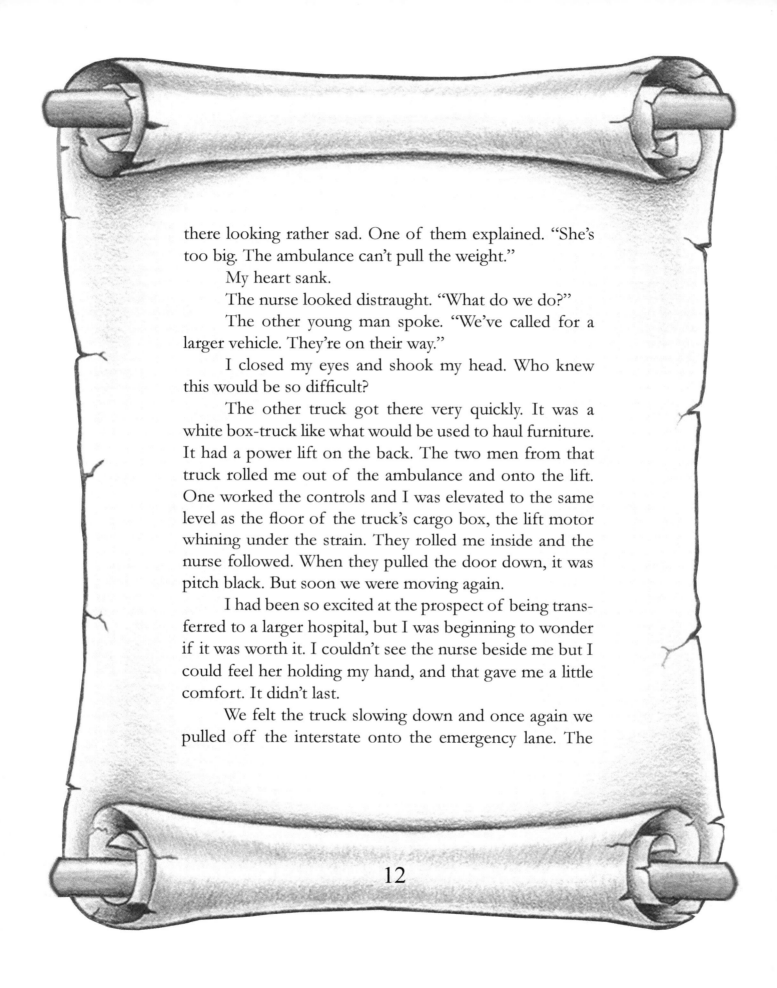

there looking rather sad. One of them explained. "She's too big. The ambulance can't pull the weight."

My heart sank.

The nurse looked distraught. "What do we do?"

The other young man spoke. "We've called for a larger vehicle. They're on their way."

I closed my eyes and shook my head. Who knew this would be so difficult?

The other truck got there very quickly. It was a white box-truck like what would be used to haul furniture. It had a power lift on the back. The two men from that truck rolled me out of the ambulance and onto the lift. One worked the controls and I was elevated to the same level as the floor of the truck's cargo box, the lift motor whining under the strain. They rolled me inside and the nurse followed. When they pulled the door down, it was pitch black. But soon we were moving again.

I had been so excited at the prospect of being transferred to a larger hospital, but I was beginning to wonder if it was worth it. I couldn't see the nurse beside me but I could feel her holding my hand, and that gave me a little comfort. It didn't last.

We felt the truck slowing down and once again we pulled off the interstate onto the emergency lane. The

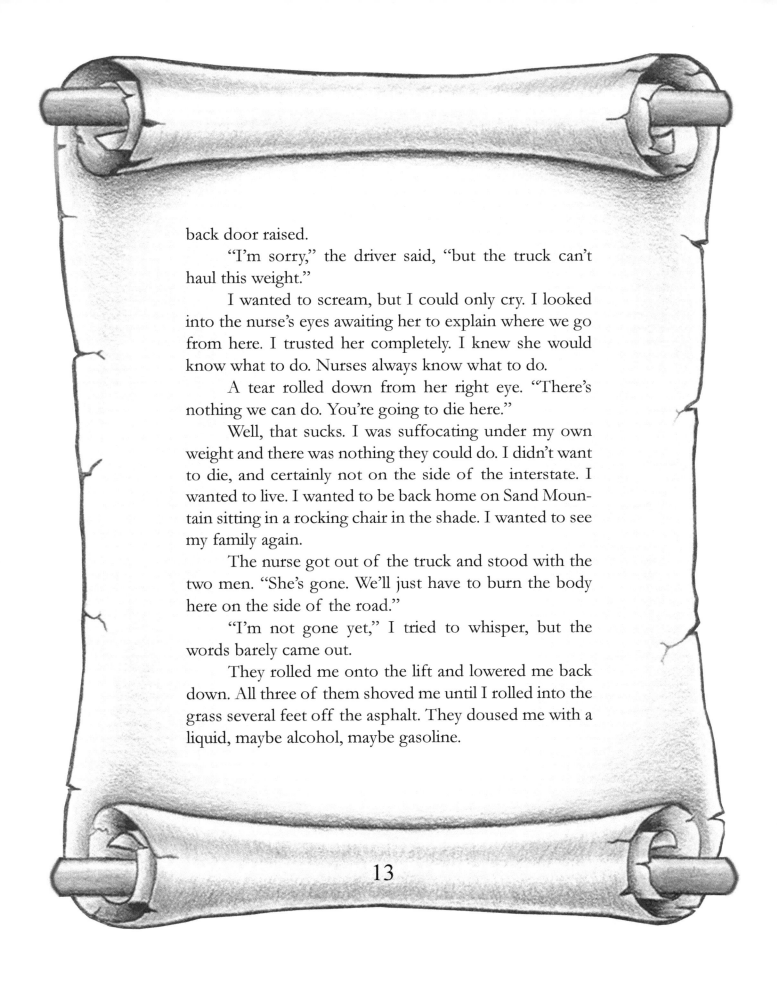

back door raised.

"I'm sorry," the driver said, "but the truck can't haul this weight."

I wanted to scream, but I could only cry. I looked into the nurse's eyes awaiting her to explain where we go from here. I trusted her completely. I knew she would know what to do. Nurses always know what to do.

A tear rolled down from her right eye. "There's nothing we can do. You're going to die here."

Well, that sucks. I was suffocating under my own weight and there was nothing they could do. I didn't want to die, and certainly not on the side of the interstate. I wanted to live. I wanted to be back home on Sand Mountain sitting in a rocking chair in the shade. I wanted to see my family again.

The nurse got out of the truck and stood with the two men. "She's gone. We'll just have to burn the body here on the side of the road."

"I'm not gone yet," I tried to whisper, but the words barely came out.

They rolled me onto the lift and lowered me back down. All three of them shoved me until I rolled into the grass several feet off the asphalt. They doused me with a liquid, maybe alcohol, maybe gasoline.

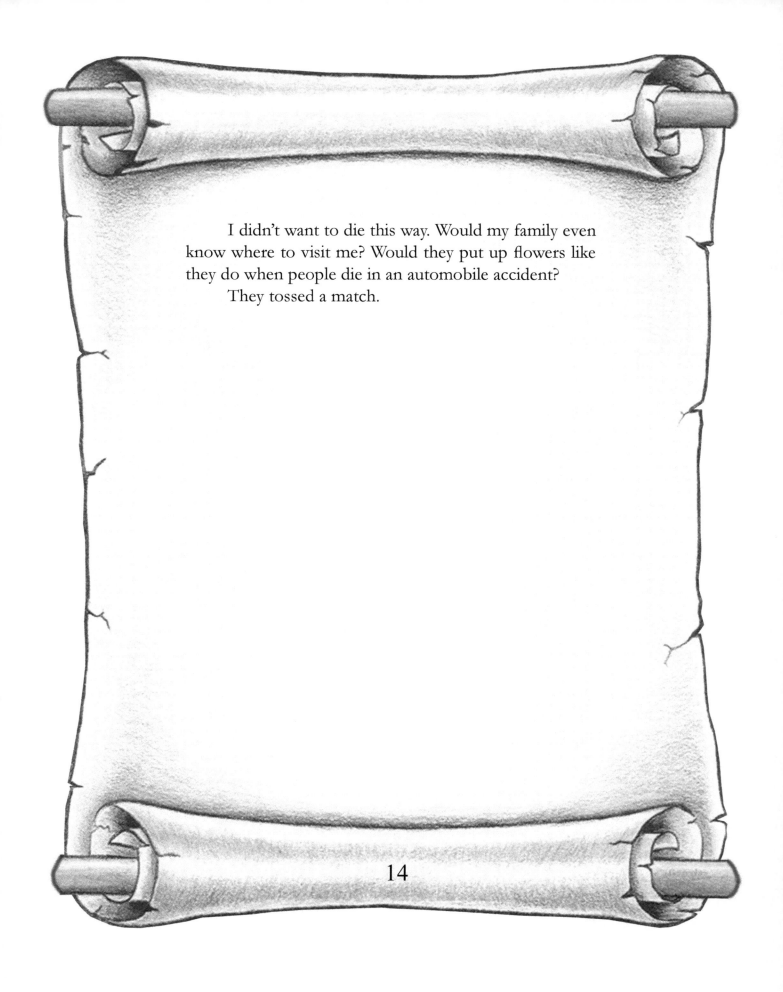

I didn't want to die this way. Would my family even know where to visit me? Would they put up flowers like they do when people die in an automobile accident?

They tossed a match.

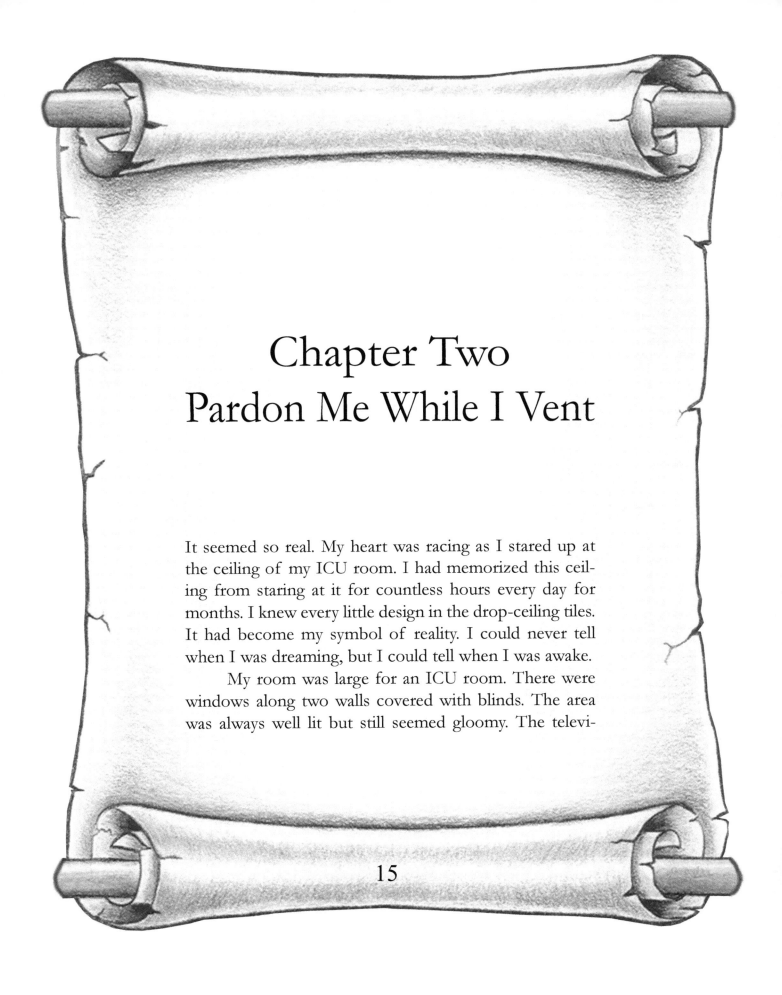

Chapter Two
Pardon Me While I Vent

It seemed so real. My heart was racing as I stared up at the ceiling of my ICU room. I had memorized this ceiling from staring at it for countless hours every day for months. I knew every little design in the drop-ceiling tiles. It had become my symbol of reality. I could never tell when I was dreaming, but I could tell when I was awake.

My room was large for an ICU room. There were windows along two walls covered with blinds. The area was always well lit but still seemed gloomy. The televi-

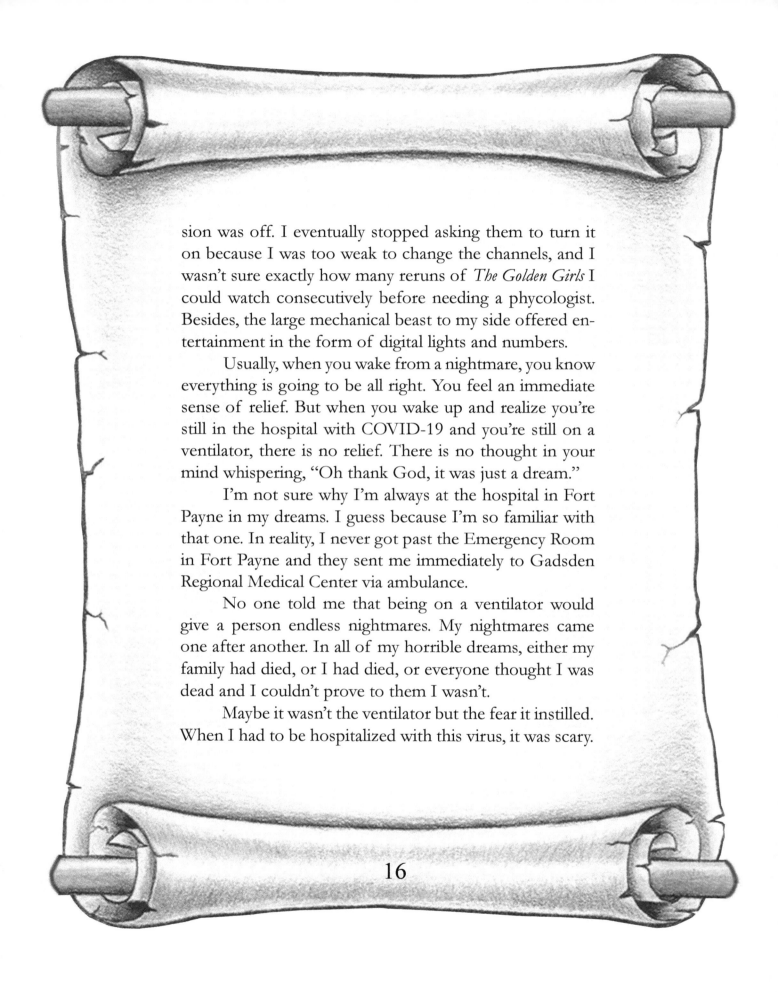

sion was off. I eventually stopped asking them to turn it on because I was too weak to change the channels, and I wasn't sure exactly how many reruns of *The Golden Girls* I could watch consecutively before needing a phycologist. Besides, the large mechanical beast to my side offered entertainment in the form of digital lights and numbers.

Usually, when you wake from a nightmare, you know everything is going to be all right. You feel an immediate sense of relief. But when you wake up and realize you're still in the hospital with COVID-19 and you're still on a ventilator, there is no relief. There is no thought in your mind whispering, "Oh thank God, it was just a dream."

I'm not sure why I'm always at the hospital in Fort Payne in my dreams. I guess because I'm so familiar with that one. In reality, I never got past the Emergency Room in Fort Payne and they sent me immediately to Gadsden Regional Medical Center via ambulance.

No one told me that being on a ventilator would give a person endless nightmares. My nightmares came one after another. In all of my horrible dreams, either my family had died, or I had died, or everyone thought I was dead and I couldn't prove to them I wasn't.

Maybe it wasn't the ventilator but the fear it instilled. When I had to be hospitalized with this virus, it was scary.

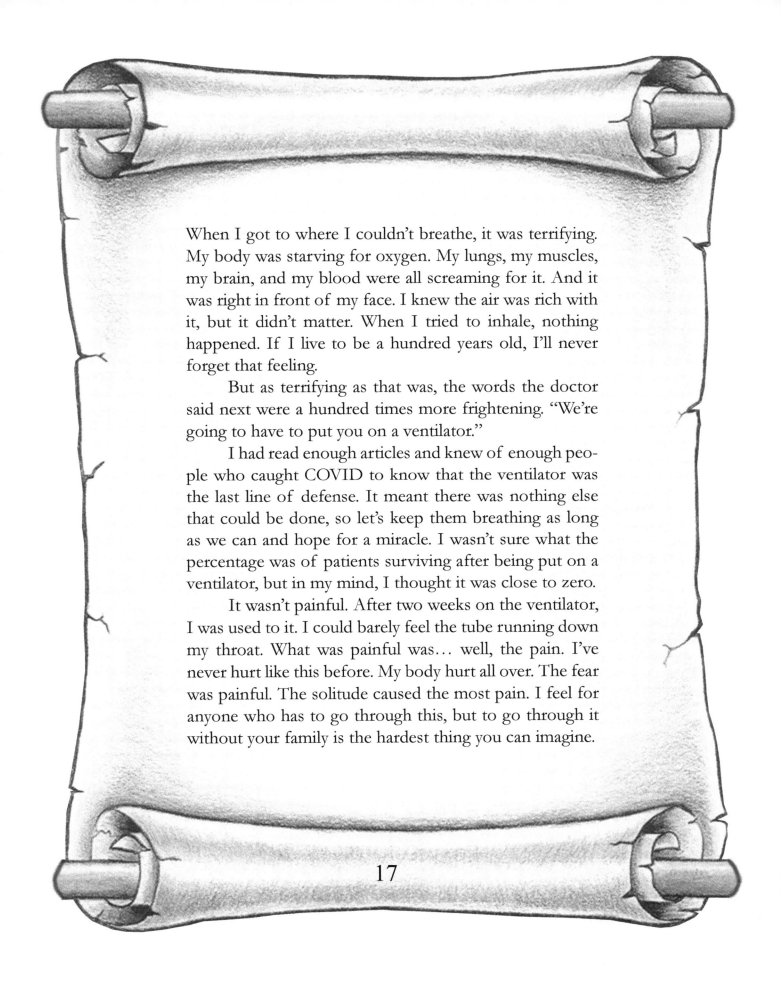

When I got to where I couldn't breathe, it was terrifying. My body was starving for oxygen. My lungs, my muscles, my brain, and my blood were all screaming for it. And it was right in front of my face. I knew the air was rich with it, but it didn't matter. When I tried to inhale, nothing happened. If I live to be a hundred years old, I'll never forget that feeling.

But as terrifying as that was, the words the doctor said next were a hundred times more frightening. "We're going to have to put you on a ventilator."

I had read enough articles and knew of enough people who caught COVID to know that the ventilator was the last line of defense. It meant there was nothing else that could be done, so let's keep them breathing as long as we can and hope for a miracle. I wasn't sure what the percentage was of patients surviving after being put on a ventilator, but in my mind, I thought it was close to zero.

It wasn't painful. After two weeks on the ventilator, I was used to it. I could barely feel the tube running down my throat. What was painful was… well, the pain. I've never hurt like this before. My body hurt all over. The fear was painful. The solitude caused the most pain. I feel for anyone who has to go through this, but to go through it without your family is the hardest thing you can imagine.

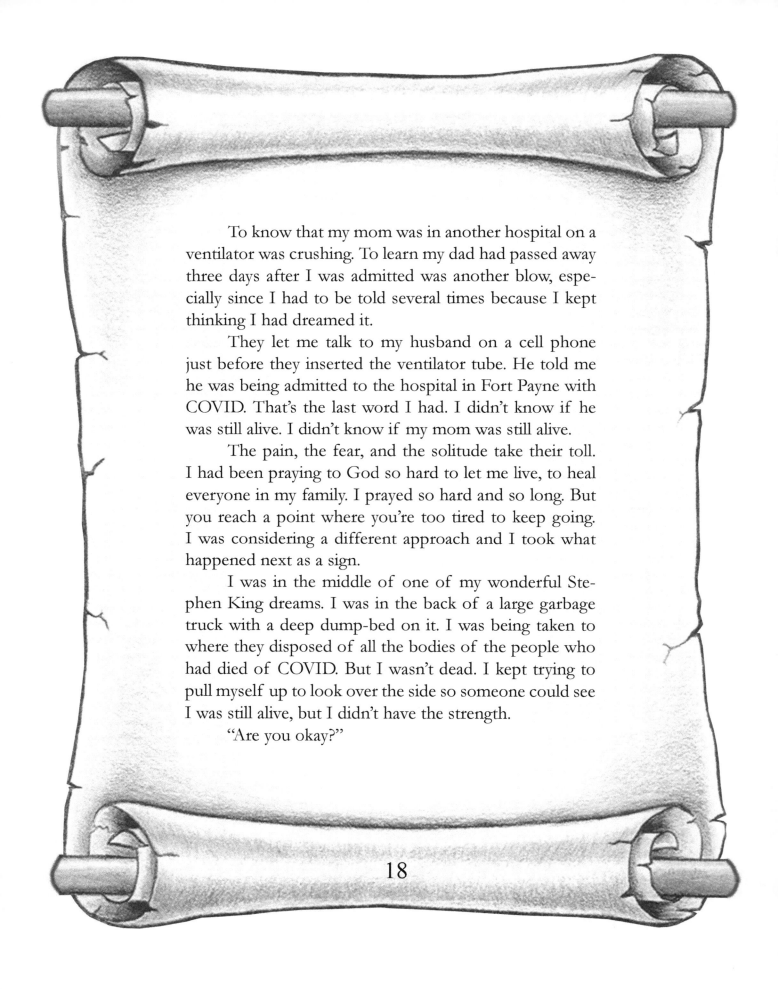

To know that my mom was in another hospital on a ventilator was crushing. To learn my dad had passed away three days after I was admitted was another blow, especially since I had to be told several times because I kept thinking I had dreamed it.

They let me talk to my husband on a cell phone just before they inserted the ventilator tube. He told me he was being admitted to the hospital in Fort Payne with COVID. That's the last word I had. I didn't know if he was still alive. I didn't know if my mom was still alive.

The pain, the fear, and the solitude take their toll. I had been praying to God so hard to let me live, to heal everyone in my family. I prayed so hard and so long. But you reach a point where you're too tired to keep going. I was considering a different approach and I took what happened next as a sign.

I was in the middle of one of my wonderful Stephen King dreams. I was in the back of a large garbage truck with a deep dump-bed on it. I was being taken to where they disposed of all the bodies of the people who had died of COVID. But I wasn't dead. I kept trying to pull myself up to look over the side so someone could see I was still alive, but I didn't have the strength.

"Are you okay?"

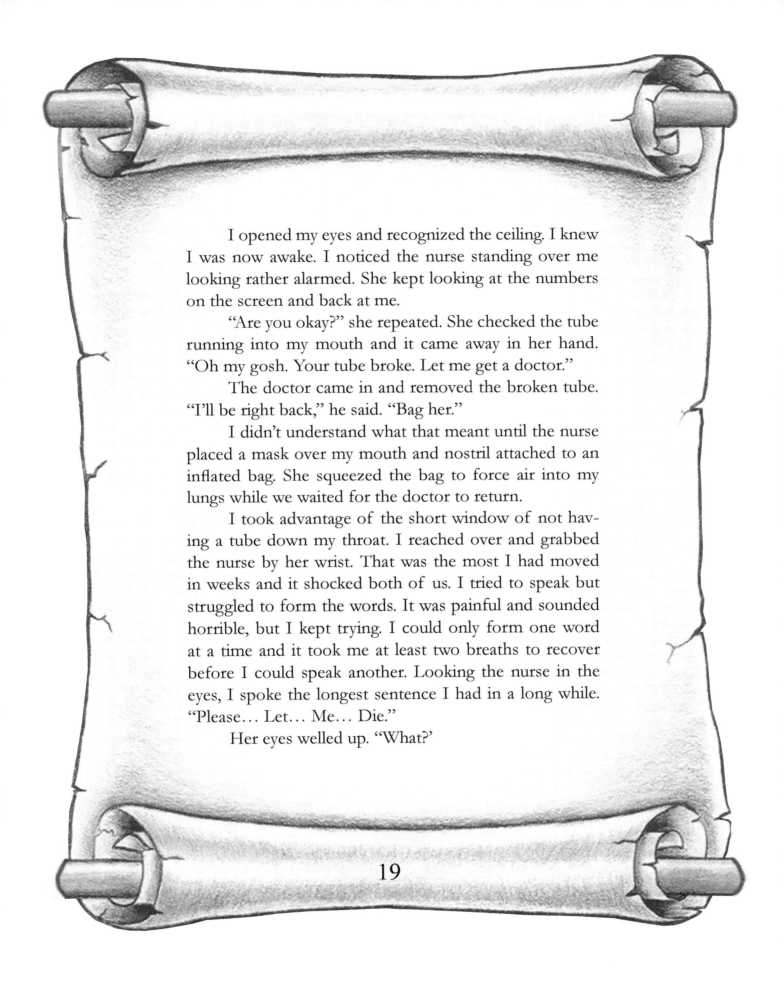

I opened my eyes and recognized the ceiling. I knew I was now awake. I noticed the nurse standing over me looking rather alarmed. She kept looking at the numbers on the screen and back at me.

"Are you okay?" she repeated. She checked the tube running into my mouth and it came away in her hand. "Oh my gosh. Your tube broke. Let me get a doctor."

The doctor came in and removed the broken tube. "I'll be right back," he said. "Bag her."

I didn't understand what that meant until the nurse placed a mask over my mouth and nostril attached to an inflated bag. She squeezed the bag to force air into my lungs while we waited for the doctor to return.

I took advantage of the short window of not having a tube down my throat. I reached over and grabbed the nurse by her wrist. That was the most I had moved in weeks and it shocked both of us. I tried to speak but struggled to form the words. It was painful and sounded horrible, but I kept trying. I could only form one word at a time and it took me at least two breaths to recover before I could speak another. Looking the nurse in the eyes, I spoke the longest sentence I had in a long while. "Please... Let... Me... Die."

Her eyes welled up. "What?'

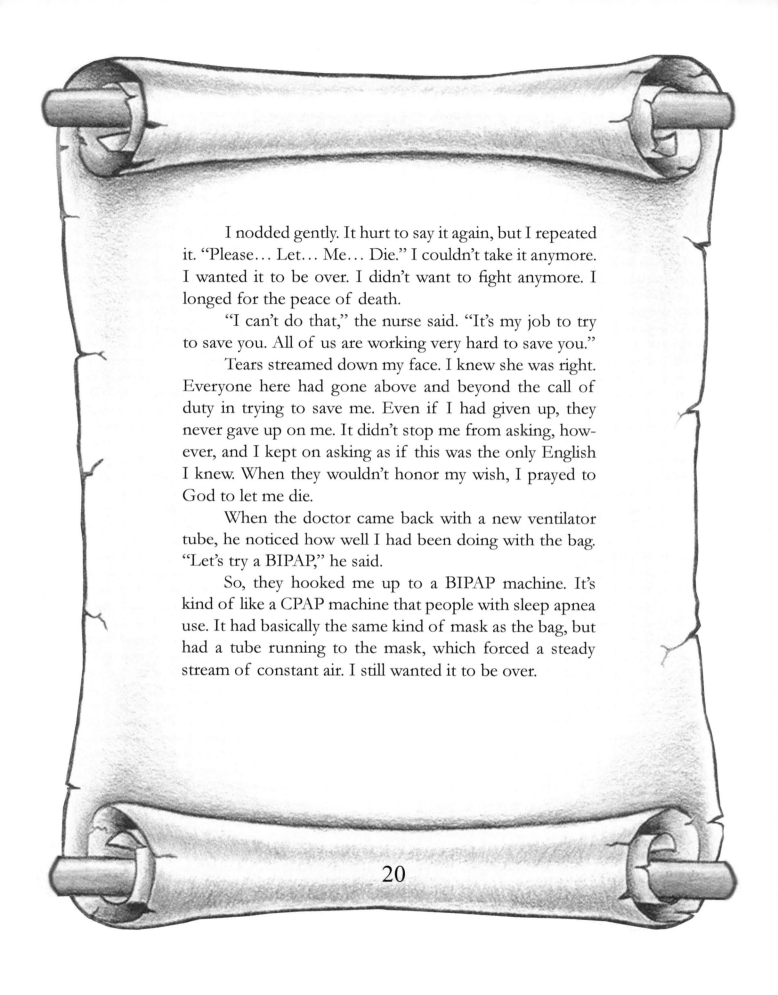

I nodded gently. It hurt to say it again, but I repeated it. "Please… Let… Me… Die." I couldn't take it anymore. I wanted it to be over. I didn't want to fight anymore. I longed for the peace of death.

"I can't do that," the nurse said. "It's my job to try to save you. All of us are working very hard to save you."

Tears streamed down my face. I knew she was right. Everyone here had gone above and beyond the call of duty in trying to save me. Even if I had given up, they never gave up on me. It didn't stop me from asking, however, and I kept on asking as if this was the only English I knew. When they wouldn't honor my wish, I prayed to God to let me die.

When the doctor came back with a new ventilator tube, he noticed how well I had been doing with the bag. "Let's try a BIPAP," he said.

So, they hooked me up to a BIPAP machine. It's kind of like a CPAP machine that people with sleep apnea use. It had basically the same kind of mask as the bag, but had a tube running to the mask, which forced a steady stream of constant air. I still wanted it to be over.

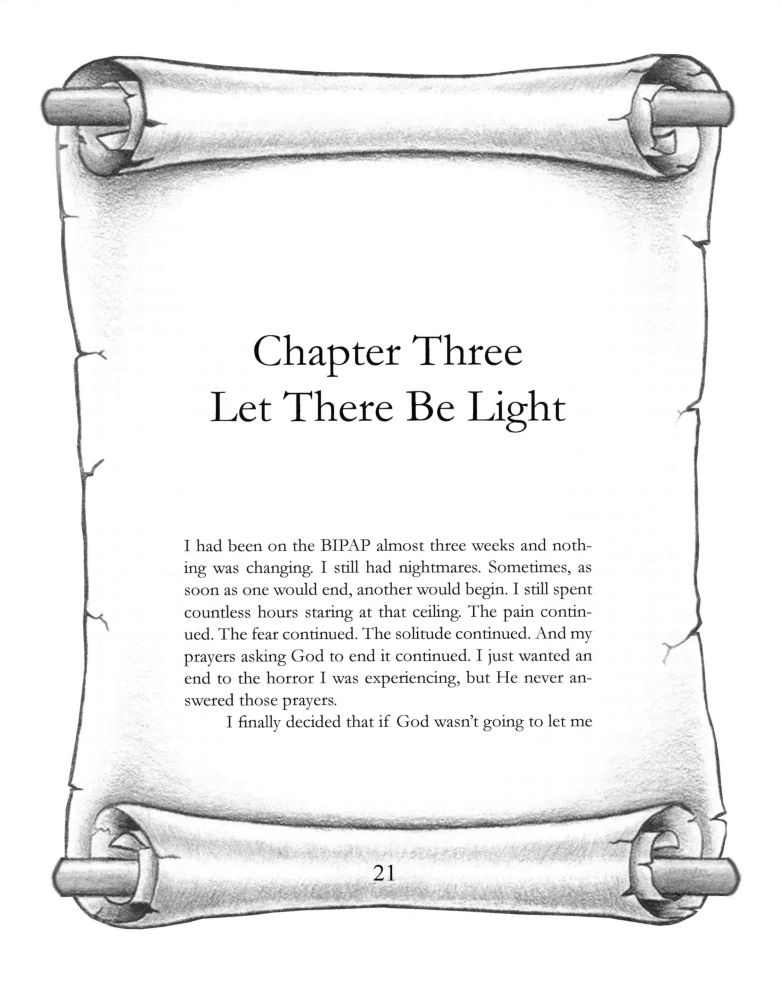

Chapter Three
Let There Be Light

I had been on the BIPAP almost three weeks and nothing was changing. I still had nightmares. Sometimes, as soon as one would end, another would begin. I still spent countless hours staring at that ceiling. The pain continued. The fear continued. The solitude continued. And my prayers asking God to end it continued. I just wanted an end to the horror I was experiencing, but He never answered those prayers.

I finally decided that if God wasn't going to let me

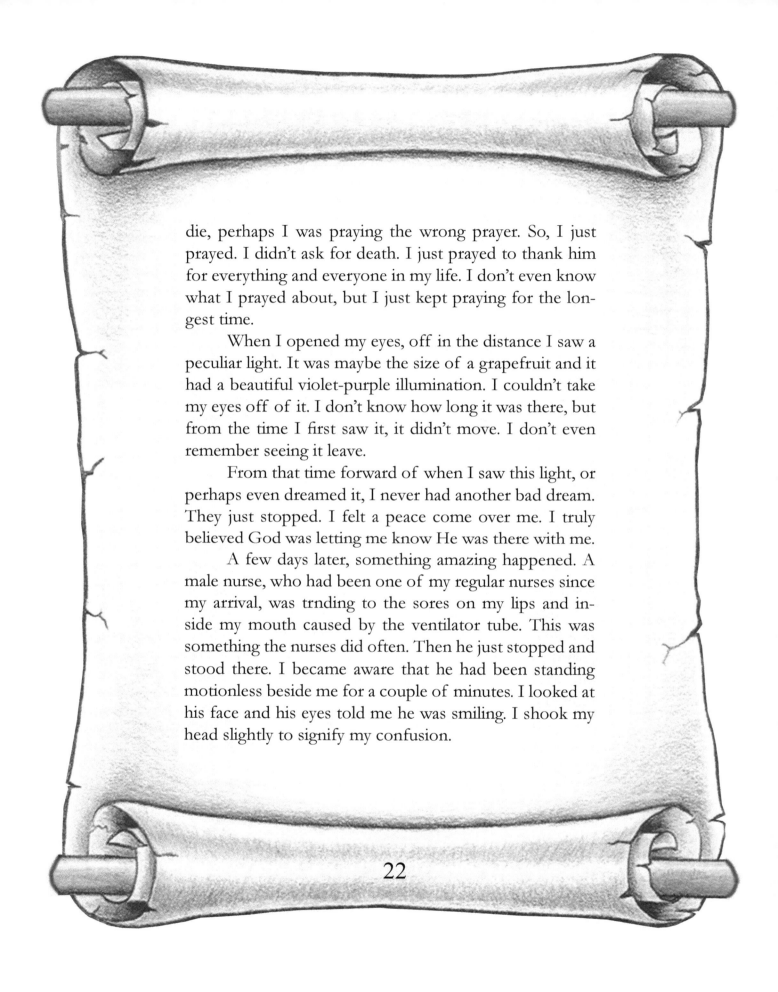

die, perhaps I was praying the wrong prayer. So, I just prayed. I didn't ask for death. I just prayed to thank him for everything and everyone in my life. I don't even know what I prayed about, but I just kept praying for the longest time.

When I opened my eyes, off in the distance I saw a peculiar light. It was maybe the size of a grapefruit and it had a beautiful violet-purple illumination. I couldn't take my eyes off of it. I don't know how long it was there, but from the time I first saw it, it didn't move. I don't even remember seeing it leave.

From that time forward of when I saw this light, or perhaps even dreamed it, I never had another bad dream. They just stopped. I felt a peace come over me. I truly believed God was letting me know He was there with me.

A few days later, something amazing happened. A male nurse, who had been one of my regular nurses since my arrival, was trnding to the sores on my lips and inside my mouth caused by the ventilator tube. This was something the nurses did often. Then he just stopped and stood there. I became aware that he had been standing motionless beside me for a couple of minutes. I looked at his face and his eyes told me he was smiling. I shook my head slightly to signify my confusion.

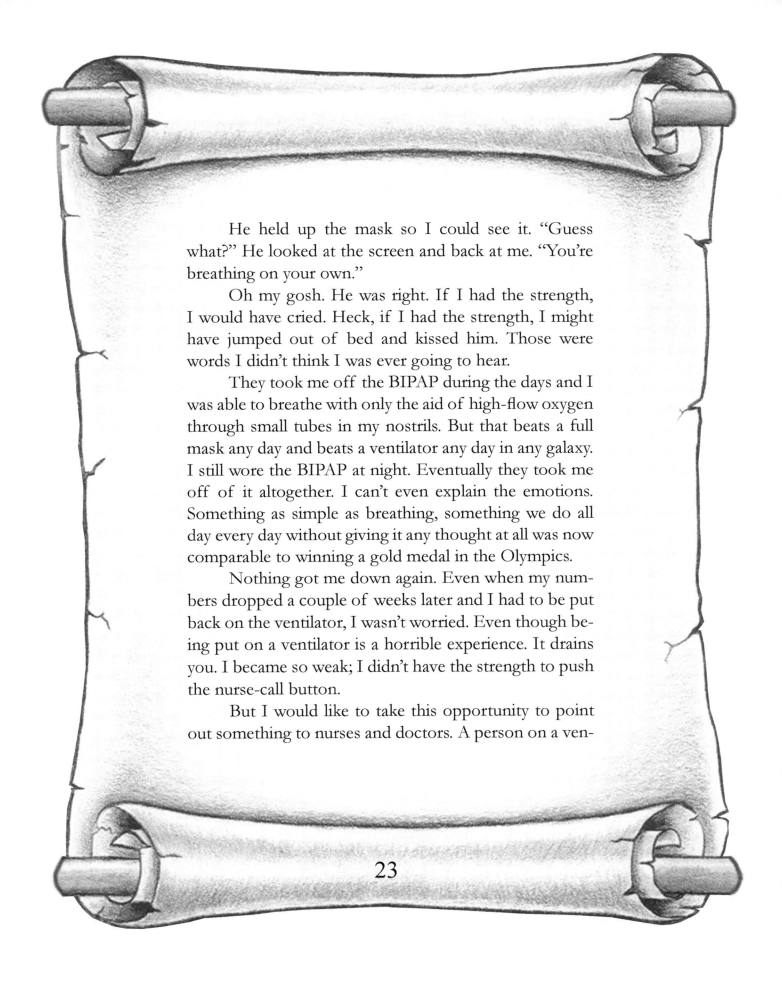

He held up the mask so I could see it. "Guess what?" He looked at the screen and back at me. "You're breathing on your own."

Oh my gosh. He was right. If I had the strength, I would have cried. Heck, if I had the strength, I might have jumped out of bed and kissed him. Those were words I didn't think I was ever going to hear.

They took me off the BIPAP during the days and I was able to breathe with only the aid of high-flow oxygen through small tubes in my nostrils. But that beats a full mask any day and beats a ventilator any day in any galaxy. I still wore the BIPAP at night. Eventually they took me off of it altogether. I can't even explain the emotions. Something as simple as breathing, something we do all day every day without giving it any thought at all was now comparable to winning a gold medal in the Olympics.

Nothing got me down again. Even when my numbers dropped a couple of weeks later and I had to be put back on the ventilator, I wasn't worried. Even though being put on a ventilator is a horrible experience. It drains you. I became so weak; I didn't have the strength to push the nurse-call button.

But I would like to take this opportunity to point out something to nurses and doctors. A person on a ven-

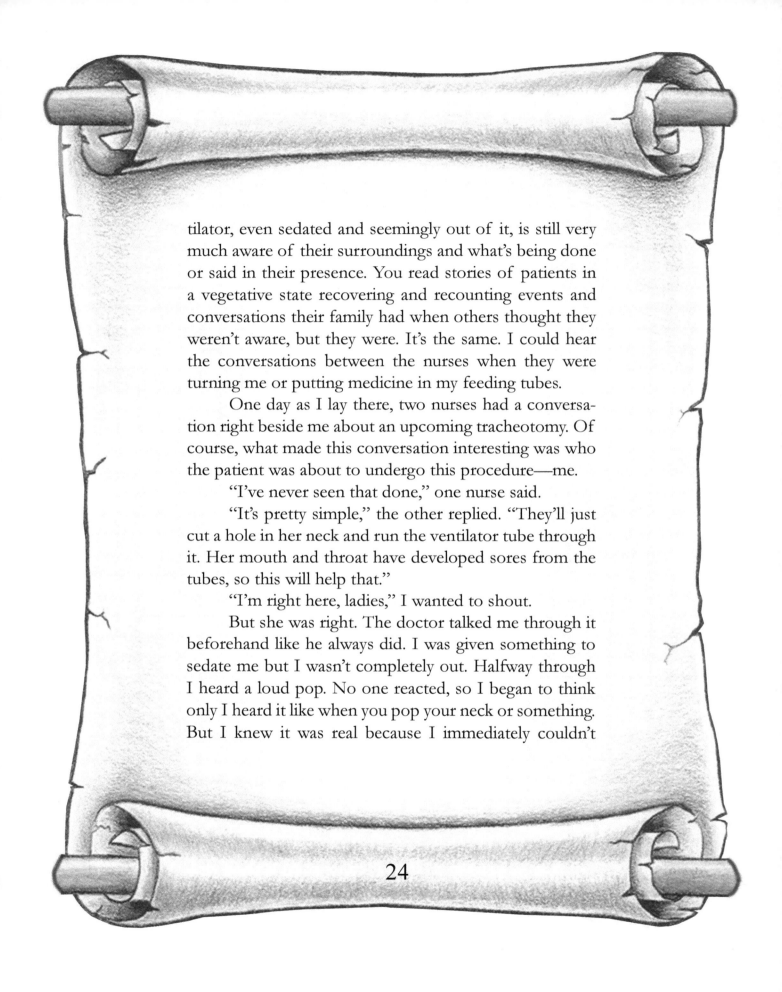

tilator, even sedated and seemingly out of it, is still very much aware of their surroundings and what's being done or said in their presence. You read stories of patients in a vegetative state recovering and recounting events and conversations their family had when others thought they weren't aware, but they were. It's the same. I could hear the conversations between the nurses when they were turning me or putting medicine in my feeding tubes.

One day as I lay there, two nurses had a conversation right beside me about an upcoming tracheotomy. Of course, what made this conversation interesting was who the patient was about to undergo this procedure—me.

"I've never seen that done," one nurse said.

"It's pretty simple," the other replied. "They'll just cut a hole in her neck and run the ventilator tube through it. Her mouth and throat have developed sores from the tubes, so this will help that."

"I'm right here, ladies," I wanted to shout.

But she was right. The doctor talked me through it beforehand like he always did. I was given something to sedate me but I wasn't completely out. Halfway through I heard a loud pop. No one reacted, so I began to think only I heard it like when you pop your neck or something. But I knew it was real because I immediately couldn't

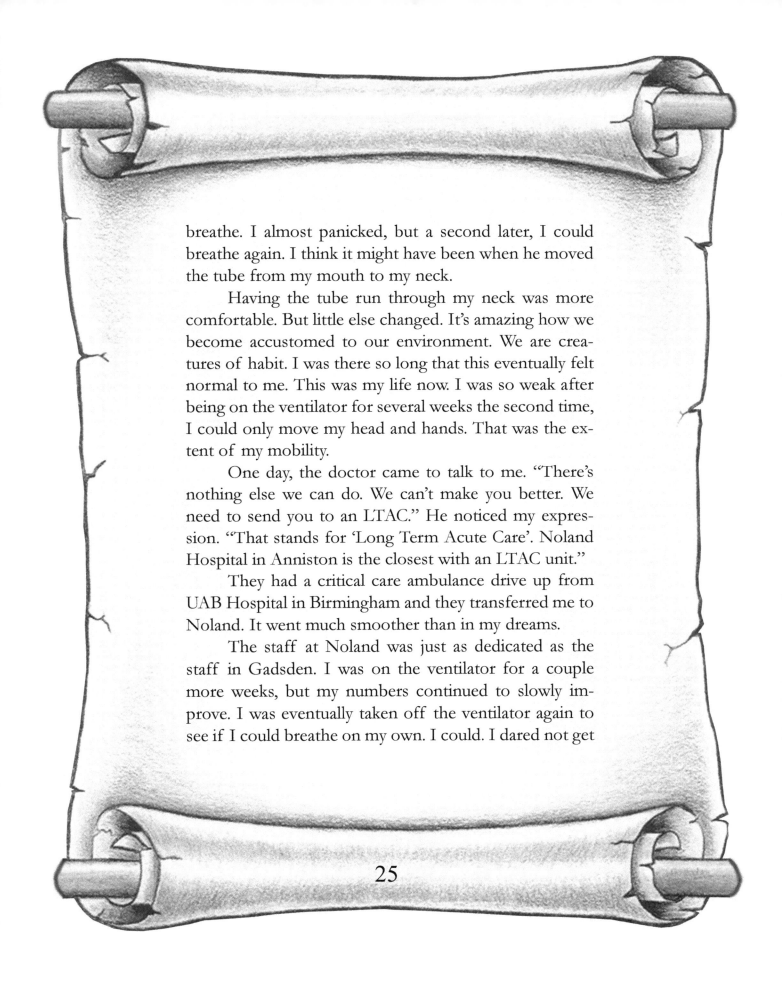

breathe. I almost panicked, but a second later, I could breathe again. I think it might have been when he moved the tube from my mouth to my neck.

Having the tube run through my neck was more comfortable. But little else changed. It's amazing how we become accustomed to our environment. We are creatures of habit. I was there so long that this eventually felt normal to me. This was my life now. I was so weak after being on the ventilator for several weeks the second time, I could only move my head and hands. That was the extent of my mobility.

One day, the doctor came to talk to me. "There's nothing else we can do. We can't make you better. We need to send you to an LTAC." He noticed my expression. "That stands for 'Long Term Acute Care'. Noland Hospital in Anniston is the closest with an LTAC unit."

They had a critical care ambulance drive up from UAB Hospital in Birmingham and they transferred me to Noland. It went much smoother than in my dreams.

The staff at Noland was just as dedicated as the staff in Gadsden. I was on the ventilator for a couple more weeks, but my numbers continued to slowly improve. I was eventually taken off the ventilator again to see if I could breathe on my own. I could. I dared not get

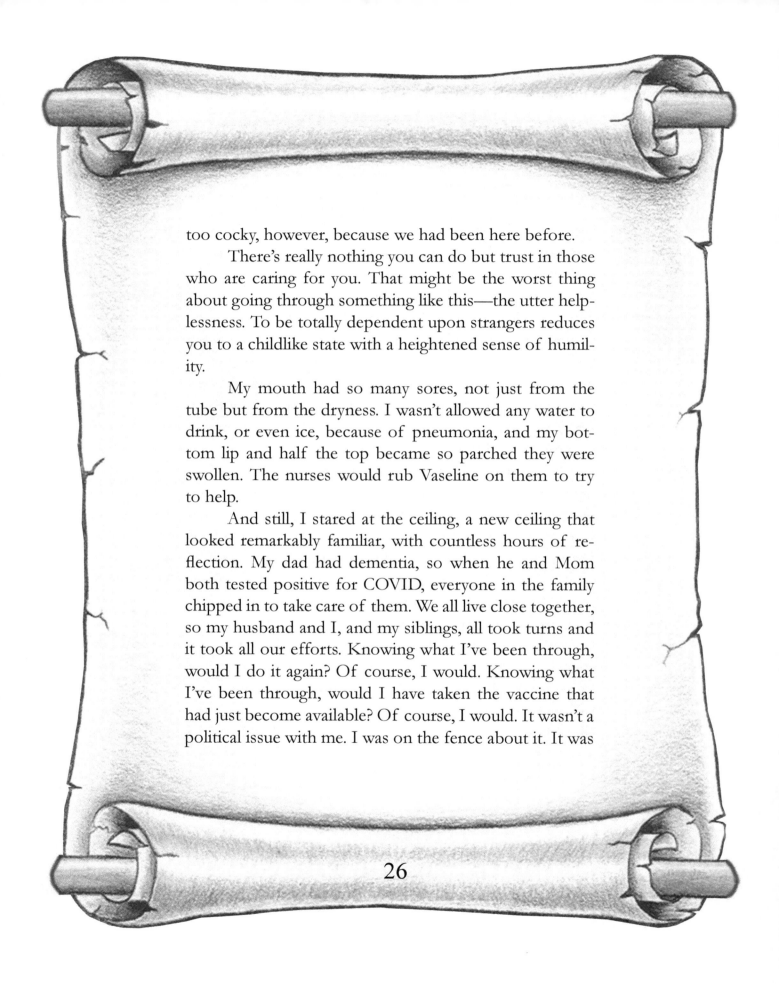

too cocky, however, because we had been here before.

There's really nothing you can do but trust in those who are caring for you. That might be the worst thing about going through something like this—the utter helplessness. To be totally dependent upon strangers reduces you to a childlike state with a heightened sense of humility.

My mouth had so many sores, not just from the tube but from the dryness. I wasn't allowed any water to drink, or even ice, because of pneumonia, and my bottom lip and half the top became so parched they were swollen. The nurses would rub Vaseline on them to try to help.

And still, I stared at the ceiling, a new ceiling that looked remarkably familiar, with countless hours of reflection. My dad had dementia, so when he and Mom both tested positive for COVID, everyone in the family chipped in to take care of them. We all live close together, so my husband and I, and my siblings, all took turns and it took all our efforts. Knowing what I've been through, would I do it again? Of course, I would. Knowing what I've been through, would I have taken the vaccine that had just become available? Of course, I would. It wasn't a political issue with me. I was on the fence about it. It was

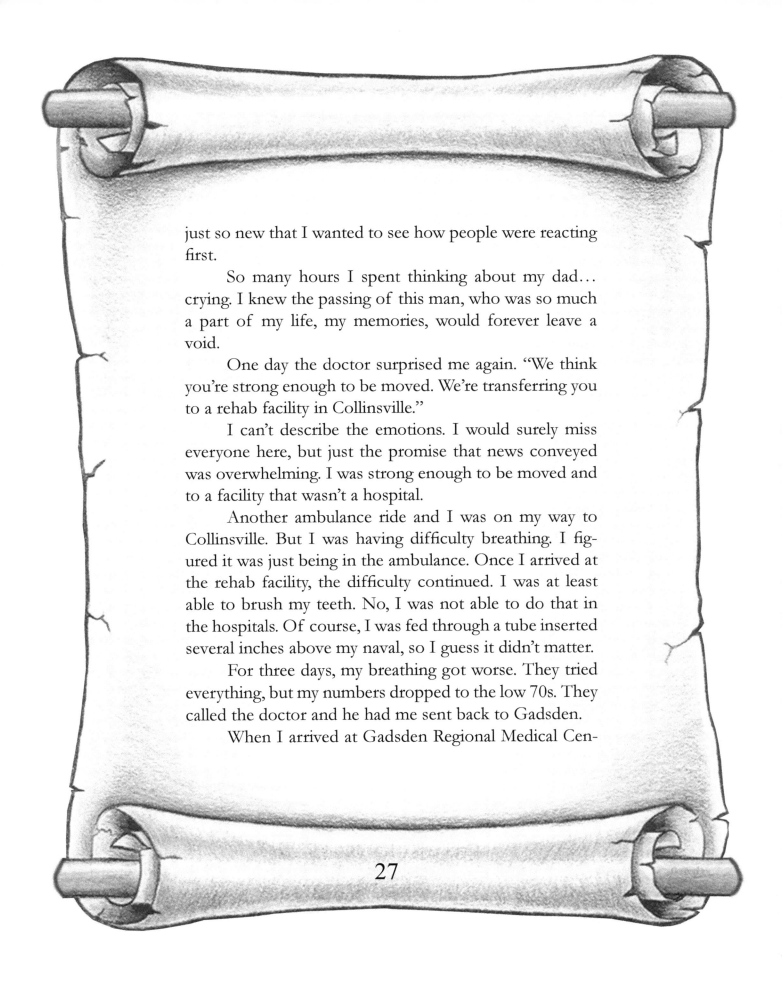

just so new that I wanted to see how people were reacting first.

So many hours I spent thinking about my dad… crying. I knew the passing of this man, who was so much a part of my life, my memories, would forever leave a void.

One day the doctor surprised me again. "We think you're strong enough to be moved. We're transferring you to a rehab facility in Collinsville."

I can't describe the emotions. I would surely miss everyone here, but just the promise that news conveyed was overwhelming. I was strong enough to be moved and to a facility that wasn't a hospital.

Another ambulance ride and I was on my way to Collinsville. But I was having difficulty breathing. I figured it was just being in the ambulance. Once I arrived at the rehab facility, the difficulty continued. I was at least able to brush my teeth. No, I was not able to do that in the hospitals. Of course, I was fed through a tube inserted several inches above my naval, so I guess it didn't matter.

For three days, my breathing got worse. They tried everything, but my numbers dropped to the low 70s. They called the doctor and he had me sent back to Gadsden.

When I arrived at Gadsden Regional Medical Cen-

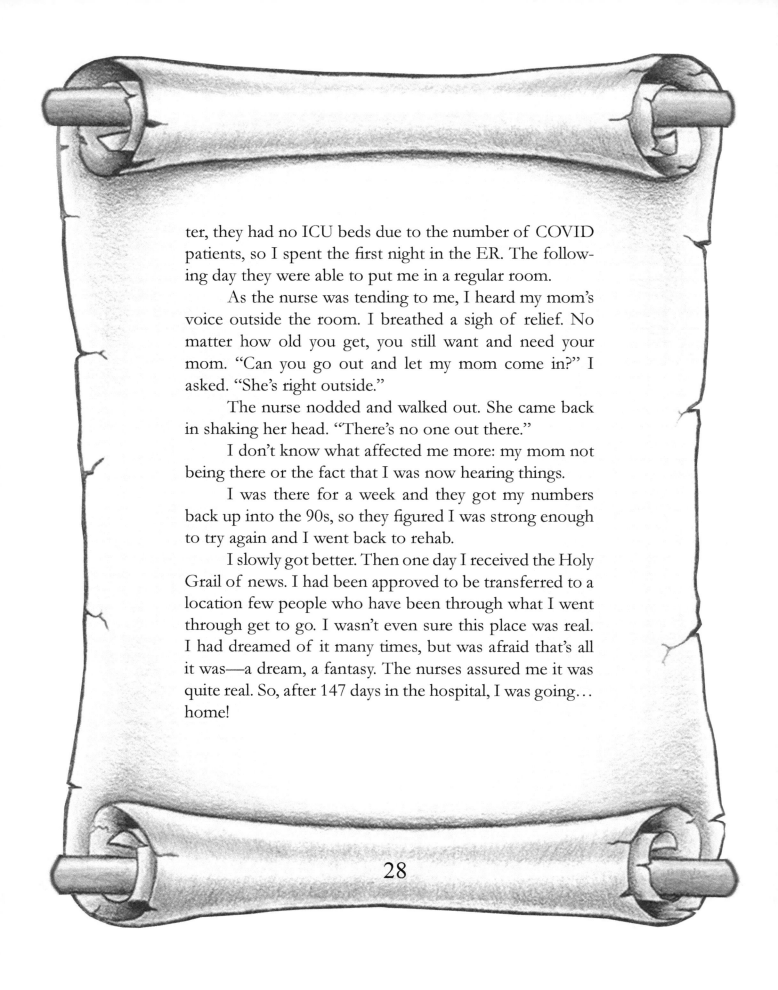

ter, they had no ICU beds due to the number of COVID patients, so I spent the first night in the ER. The following day they were able to put me in a regular room.

As the nurse was tending to me, I heard my mom's voice outside the room. I breathed a sigh of relief. No matter how old you get, you still want and need your mom. "Can you go out and let my mom come in?" I asked. "She's right outside."

The nurse nodded and walked out. She came back in shaking her head. "There's no one out there."

I don't know what affected me more: my mom not being there or the fact that I was now hearing things.

I was there for a week and they got my numbers back up into the 90s, so they figured I was strong enough to try again and I went back to rehab.

I slowly got better. Then one day I received the Holy Grail of news. I had been approved to be transferred to a location few people who have been through what I went through get to go. I wasn't even sure this place was real. I had dreamed of it many times, but was afraid that's all it was—a dream, a fantasy. The nurses assured me it was quite real. So, after 147 days in the hospital, I was going… home!

Chapter Four
No Place Like Home

My husband rolled me to the center of our living room and I soaked it in.

"What do you want to do first?" he asked.

"Go to bed."

He laughed. "After all the time you've spent in bed the last few months?"

I know it sounded terrible, but I was drained.

"You feel like sitting on the front porch?" he asked.

I nodded. "Sure."

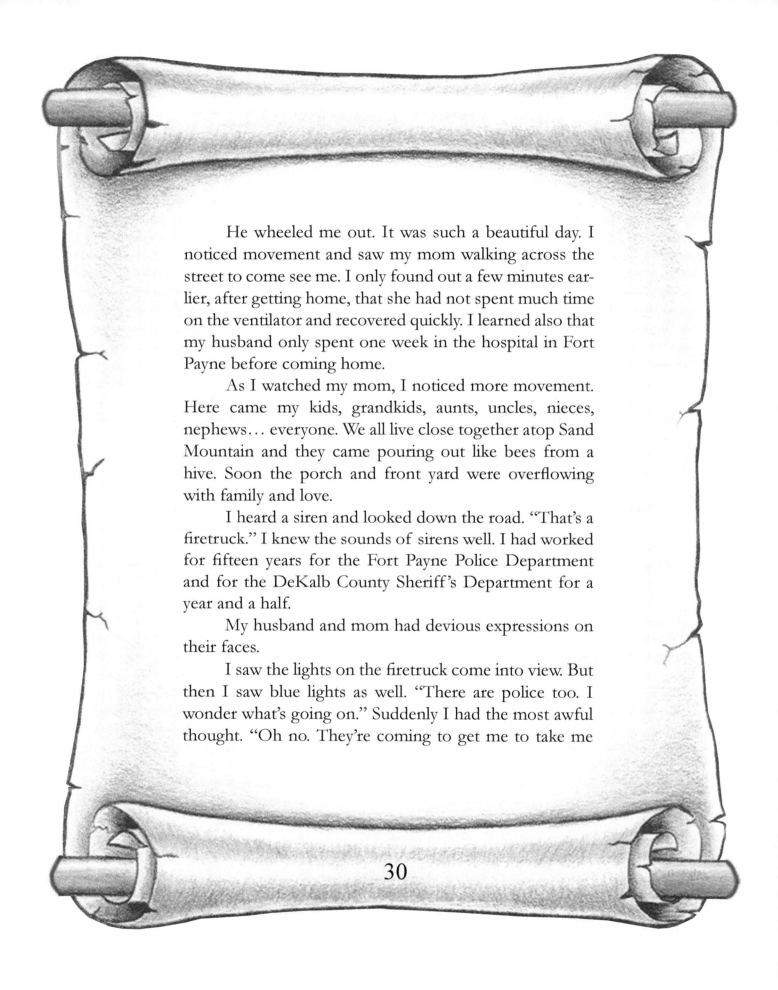

He wheeled me out. It was such a beautiful day. I noticed movement and saw my mom walking across the street to come see me. I only found out a few minutes earlier, after getting home, that she had not spent much time on the ventilator and recovered quickly. I learned also that my husband only spent one week in the hospital in Fort Payne before coming home.

As I watched my mom, I noticed more movement. Here came my kids, grandkids, aunts, uncles, nieces, nephews... everyone. We all live close together atop Sand Mountain and they came pouring out like bees from a hive. Soon the porch and front yard were overflowing with family and love.

I heard a siren and looked down the road. "That's a firetruck." I knew the sounds of sirens well. I had worked for fifteen years for the Fort Payne Police Department and for the DeKalb County Sheriff's Department for a year and a half.

My husband and mom had devious expressions on their faces.

I saw the lights on the firetruck come into view. But then I saw blue lights as well. "There are police too. I wonder what's going on." Suddenly I had the most awful thought. "Oh no. They're coming to get me to take me

30

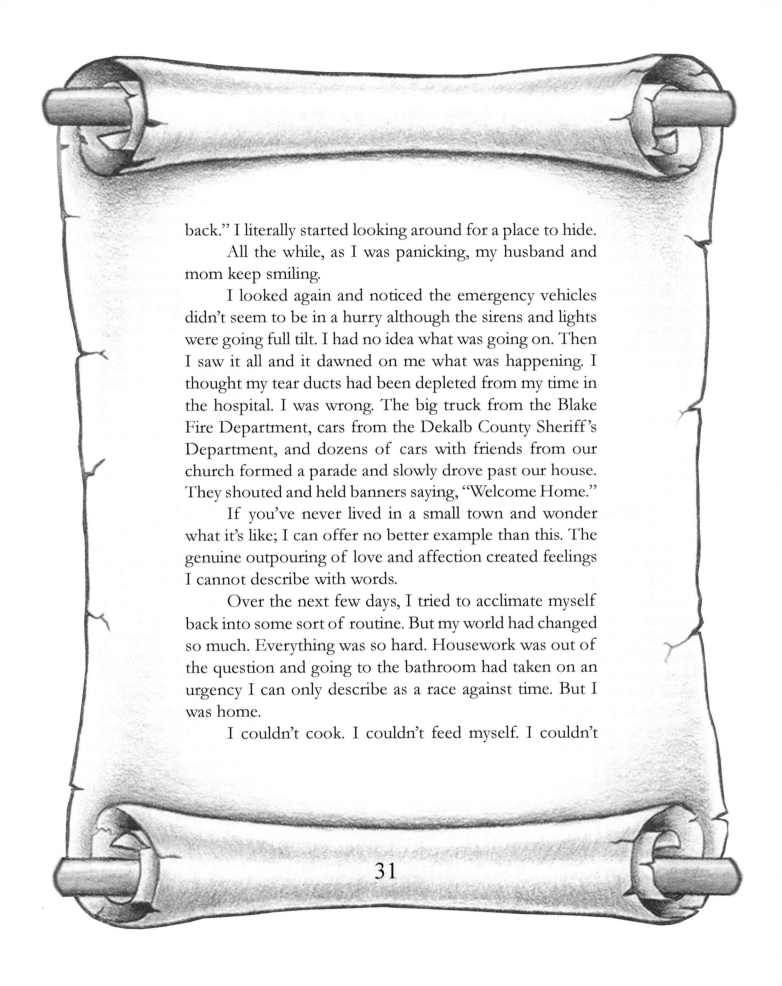

back." I literally started looking around for a place to hide.

All the while, as I was panicking, my husband and mom keep smiling.

I looked again and noticed the emergency vehicles didn't seem to be in a hurry although the sirens and lights were going full tilt. I had no idea what was going on. Then I saw it all and it dawned on me what was happening. I thought my tear ducts had been depleted from my time in the hospital. I was wrong. The big truck from the Blake Fire Department, cars from the Dekalb County Sheriff's Department, and dozens of cars with friends from our church formed a parade and slowly drove past our house. They shouted and held banners saying, "Welcome Home."

If you've never lived in a small town and wonder what it's like; I can offer no better example than this. The genuine outpouring of love and affection created feelings I cannot describe with words.

Over the next few days, I tried to acclimate myself back into some sort of routine. But my world had changed so much. Everything was so hard. Housework was out of the question and going to the bathroom had taken on an urgency I can only describe as a race against time. But I was home.

I couldn't cook. I couldn't feed myself. I couldn't

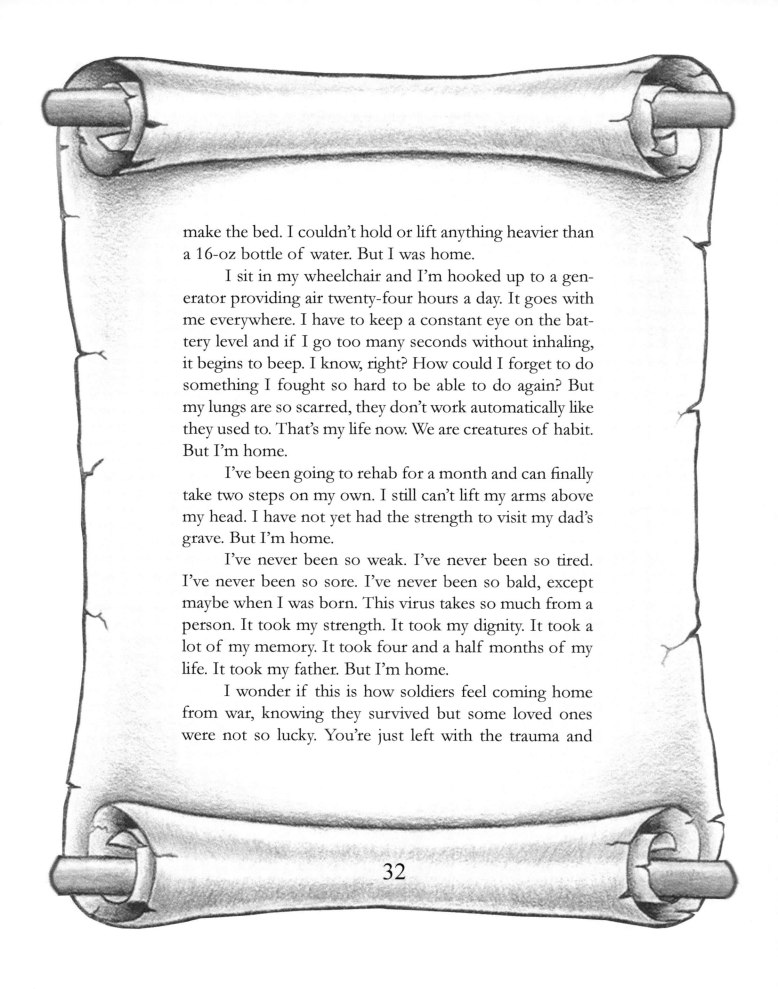

make the bed. I couldn't hold or lift anything heavier than a 16-oz bottle of water. But I was home.

I sit in my wheelchair and I'm hooked up to a generator providing air twenty-four hours a day. It goes with me everywhere. I have to keep a constant eye on the battery level and if I go too many seconds without inhaling, it begins to beep. I know, right? How could I forget to do something I fought so hard to be able to do again? But my lungs are so scarred, they don't work automatically like they used to. That's my life now. We are creatures of habit. But I'm home.

I've been going to rehab for a month and can finally take two steps on my own. I still can't lift my arms above my head. I have not yet had the strength to visit my dad's grave. But I'm home.

I've never been so weak. I've never been so tired. I've never been so sore. I've never been so bald, except maybe when I was born. This virus takes so much from a person. It took my strength. It took my dignity. It took a lot of my memory. It took four and a half months of my life. It took my father. But I'm home.

I wonder if this is how soldiers feel coming home from war, knowing they survived but some loved ones were not so lucky. You're just left with the trauma and

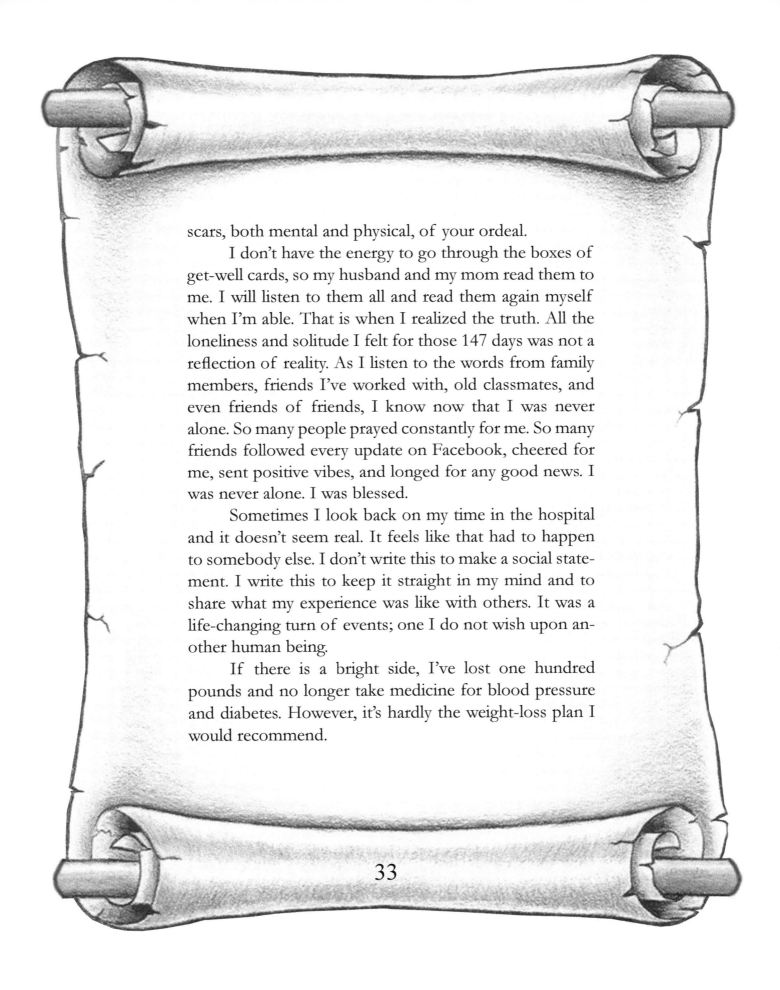

scars, both mental and physical, of your ordeal.

I don't have the energy to go through the boxes of get-well cards, so my husband and my mom read them to me. I will listen to them all and read them again myself when I'm able. That is when I realized the truth. All the loneliness and solitude I felt for those 147 days was not a reflection of reality. As I listen to the words from family members, friends I've worked with, old classmates, and even friends of friends, I know now that I was never alone. So many people prayed constantly for me. So many friends followed every update on Facebook, cheered for me, sent positive vibes, and longed for any good news. I was never alone. I was blessed.

Sometimes I look back on my time in the hospital and it doesn't seem real. It feels like that had to happen to somebody else. I don't write this to make a social statement. I write this to keep it straight in my mind and to share what my experience was like with others. It was a life-changing turn of events; one I do not wish upon another human being.

If there is a bright side, I've lost one hundred pounds and no longer take medicine for blood pressure and diabetes. However, it's hardly the weight-loss plan I would recommend.

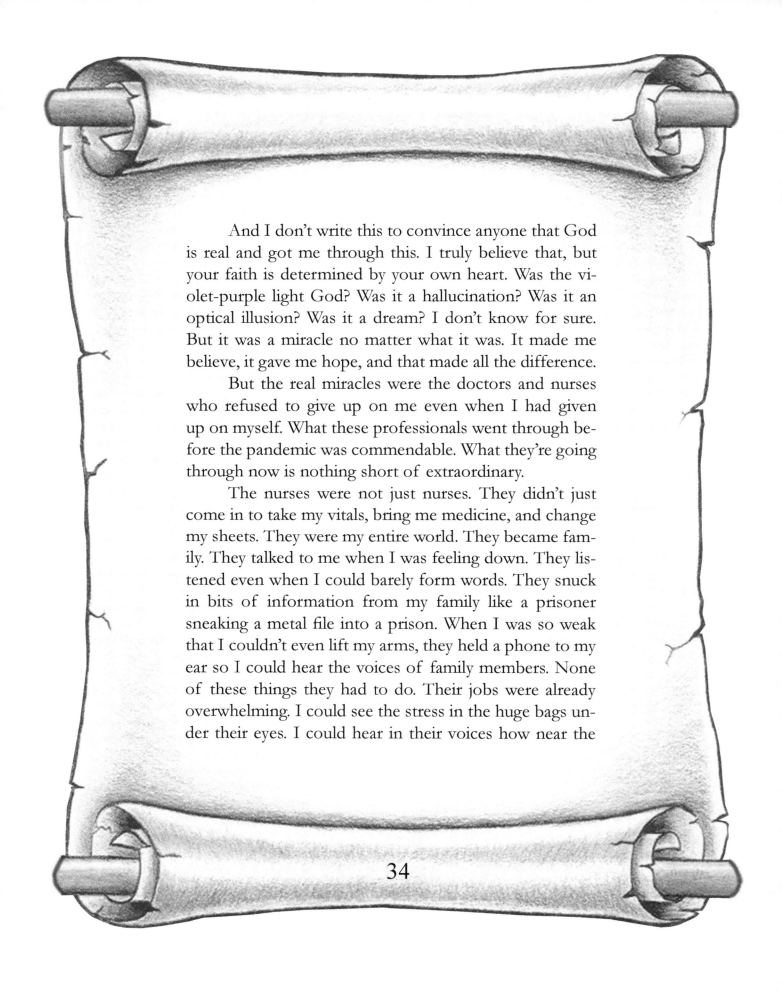

And I don't write this to convince anyone that God is real and got me through this. I truly believe that, but your faith is determined by your own heart. Was the violet-purple light God? Was it a hallucination? Was it an optical illusion? Was it a dream? I don't know for sure. But it was a miracle no matter what it was. It made me believe, it gave me hope, and that made all the difference.

But the real miracles were the doctors and nurses who refused to give up on me even when I had given up on myself. What these professionals went through before the pandemic was commendable. What they're going through now is nothing short of extraordinary.

The nurses were not just nurses. They didn't just come in to take my vitals, bring me medicine, and change my sheets. They were my entire world. They became family. They talked to me when I was feeling down. They listened even when I could barely form words. They snuck in bits of information from my family like a prisoner sneaking a metal file into a prison. When I was so weak that I couldn't even lift my arms, they held a phone to my ear so I could hear the voices of family members. None of these things they had to do. Their jobs were already overwhelming. I could see the stress in the huge bags under their eyes. I could hear in their voices how near the

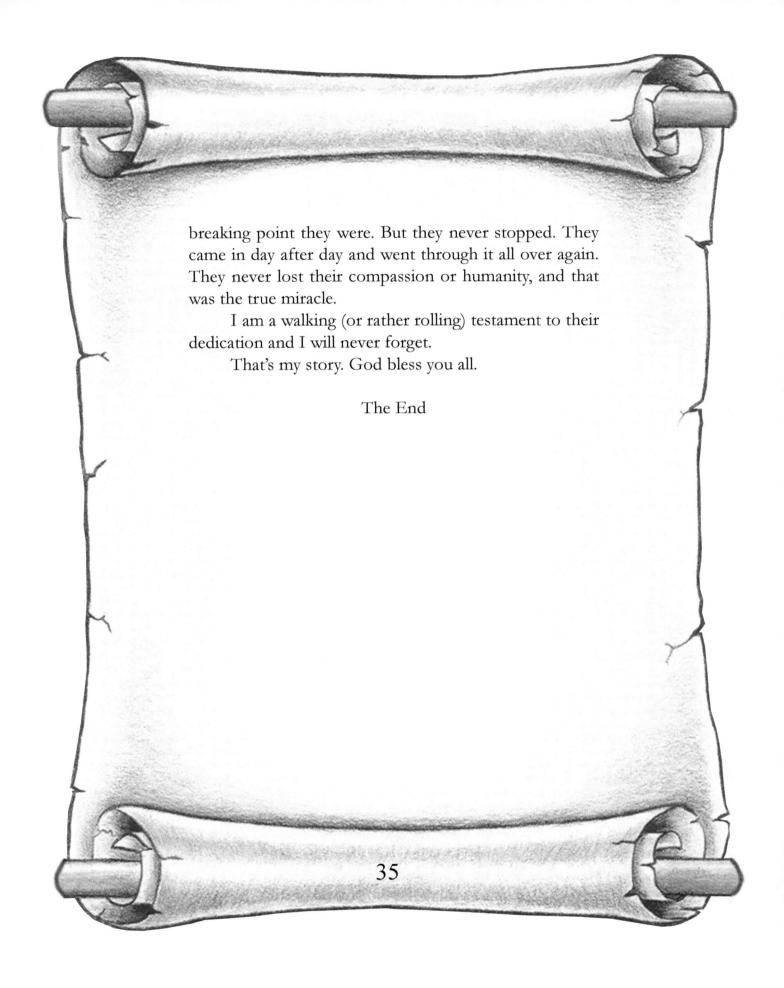

breaking point they were. But they never stopped. They came in day after day and went through it all over again. They never lost their compassion or humanity, and that was the true miracle.

I am a walking (or rather rolling) testament to their dedication and I will never forget.

That's my story. God bless you all.

The End

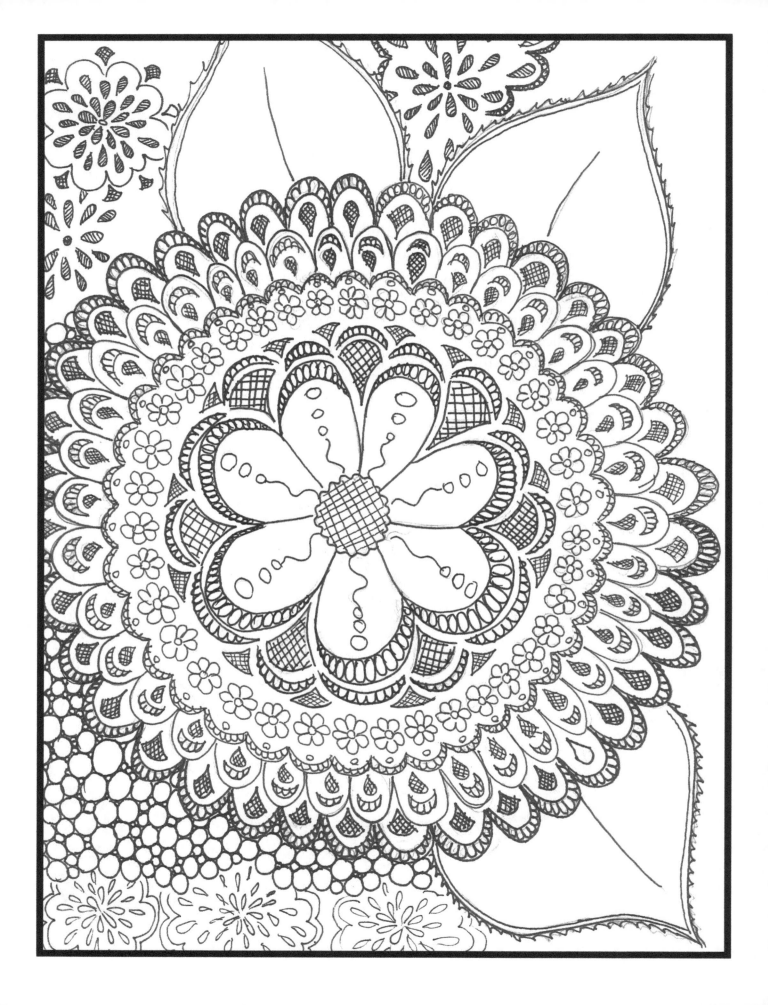

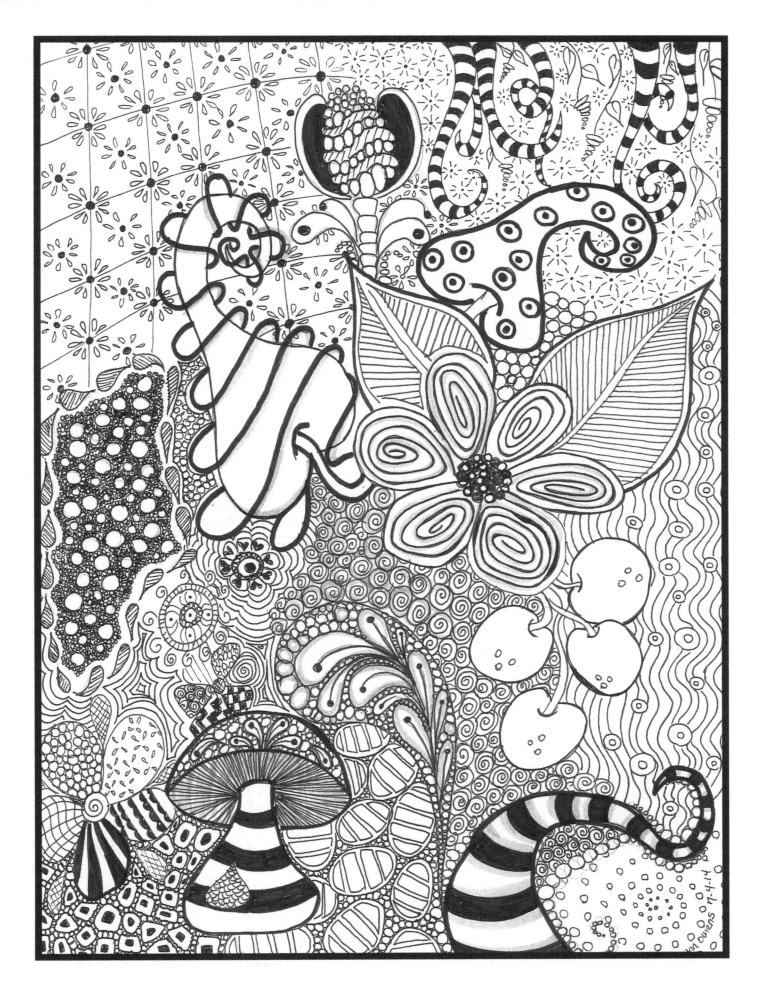

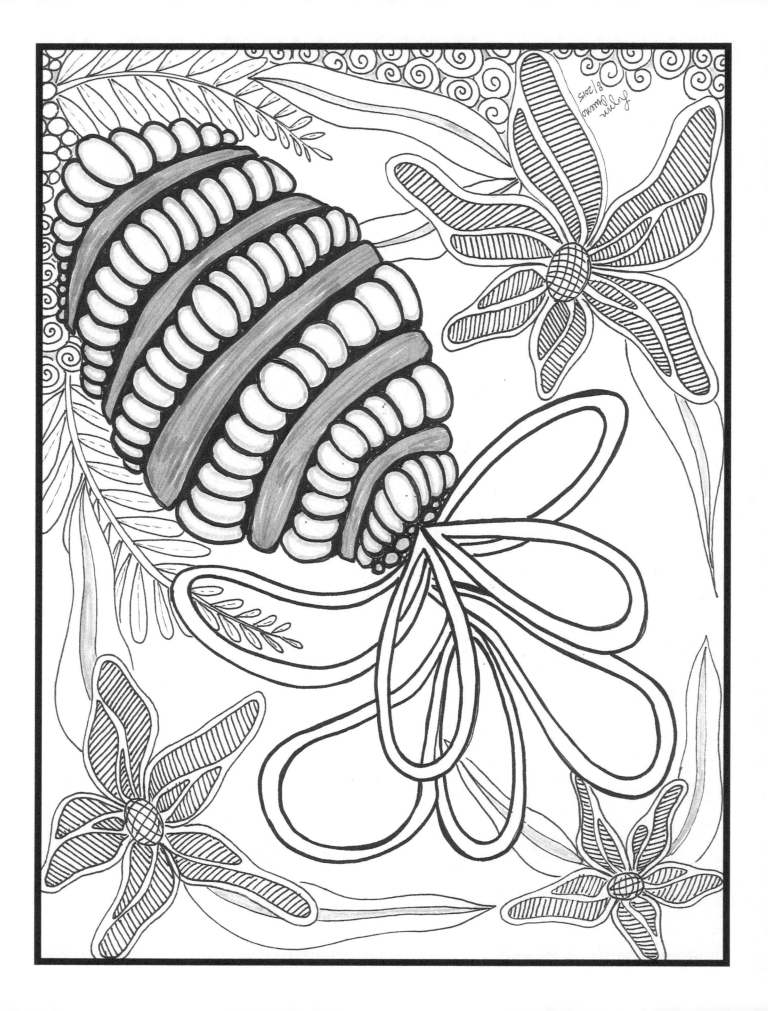

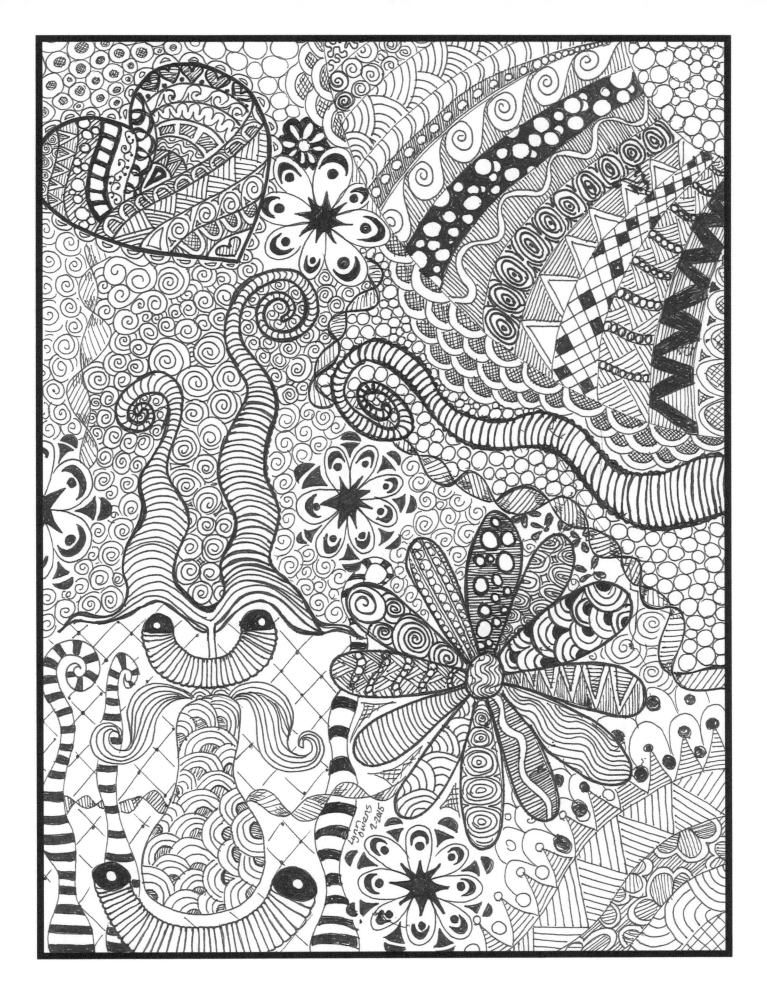

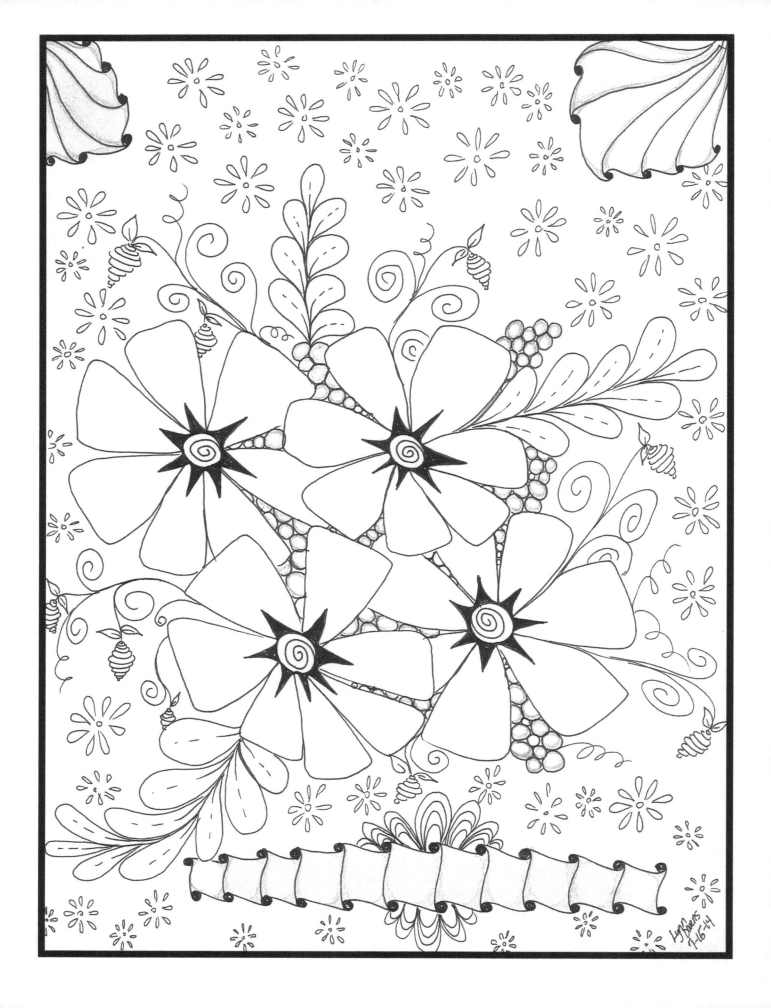

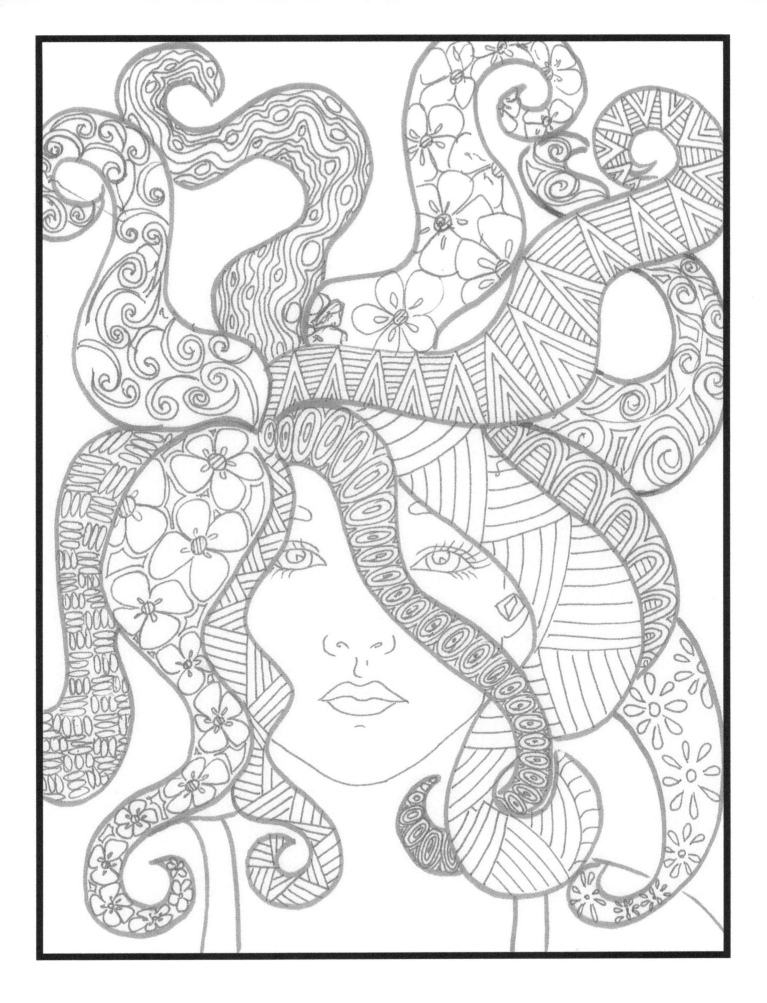

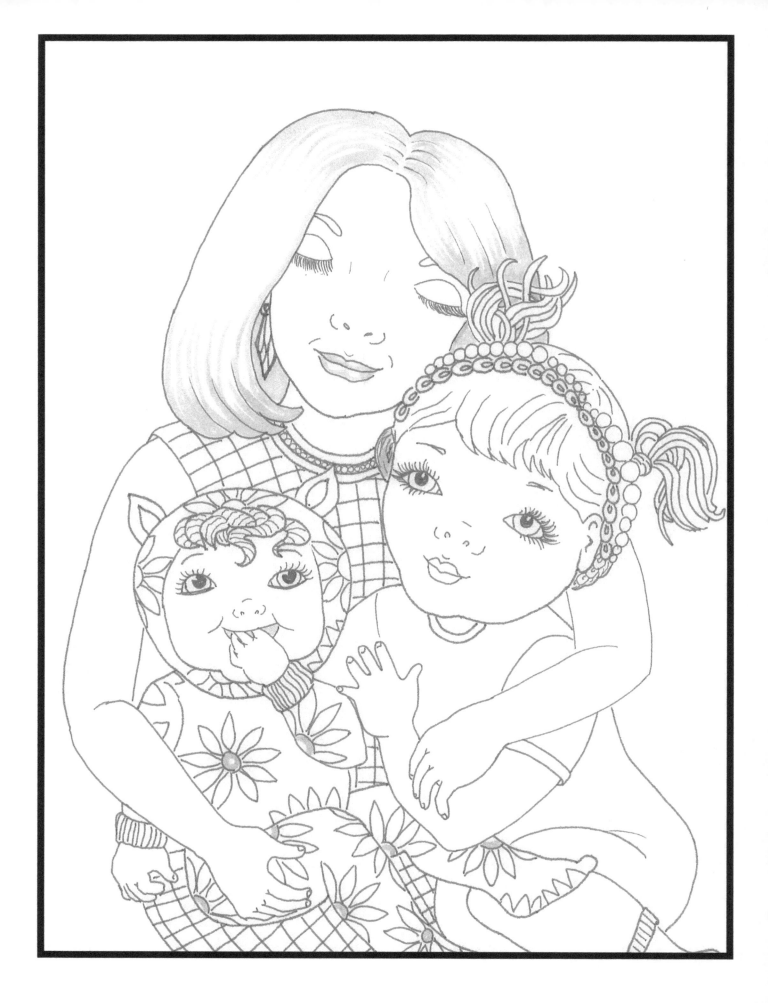

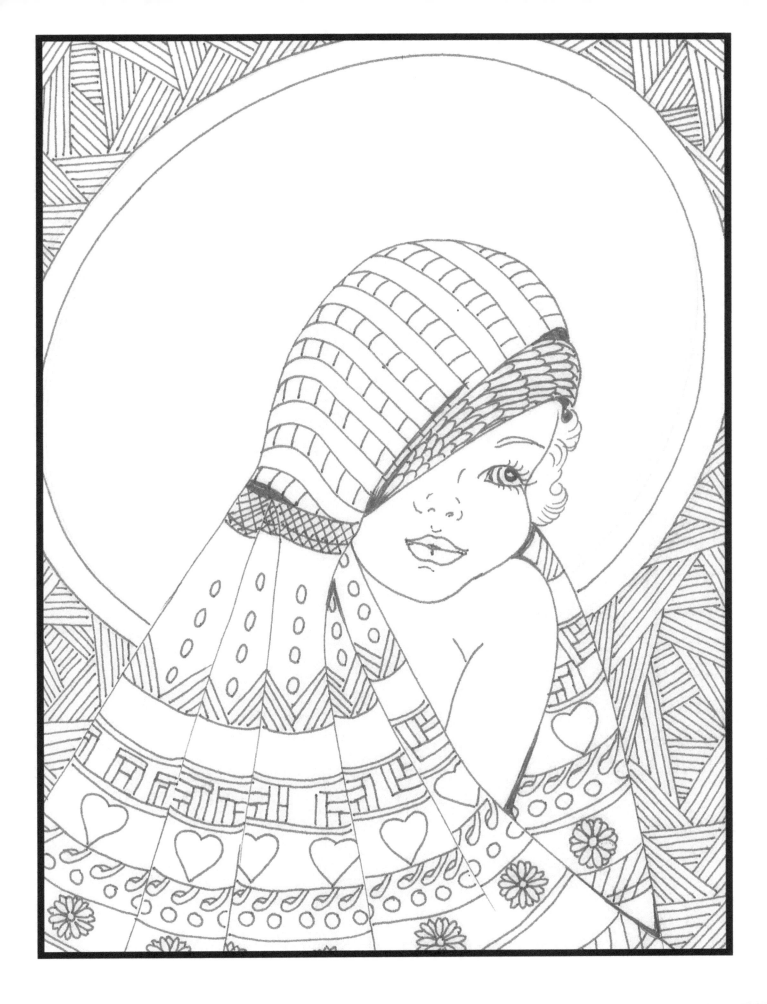

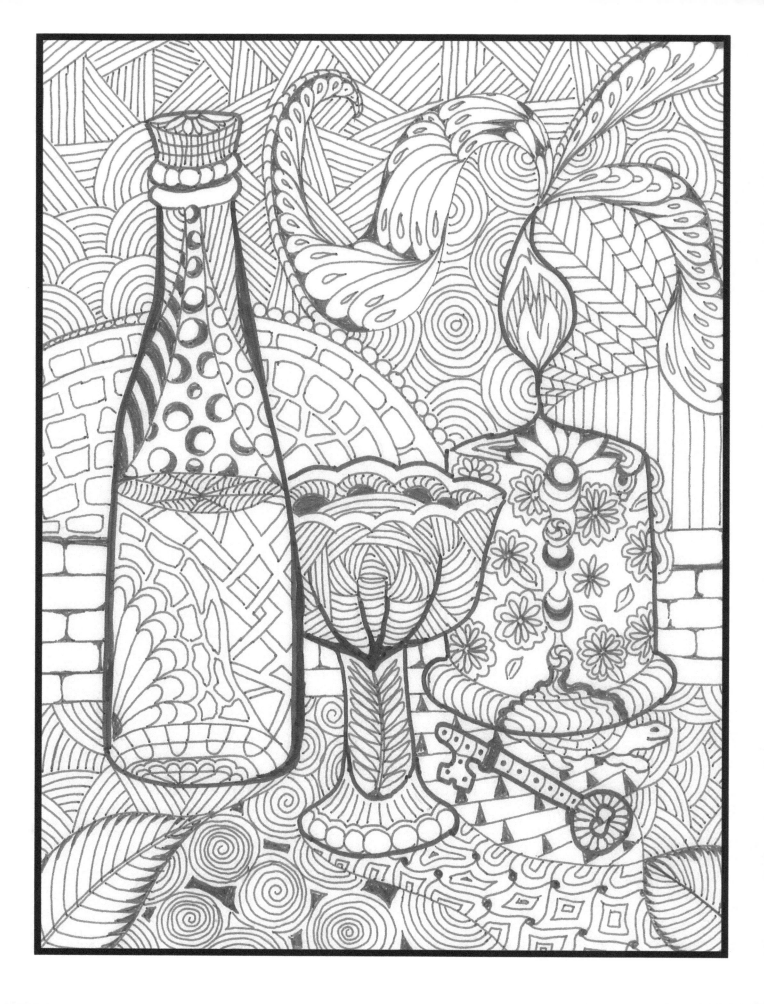

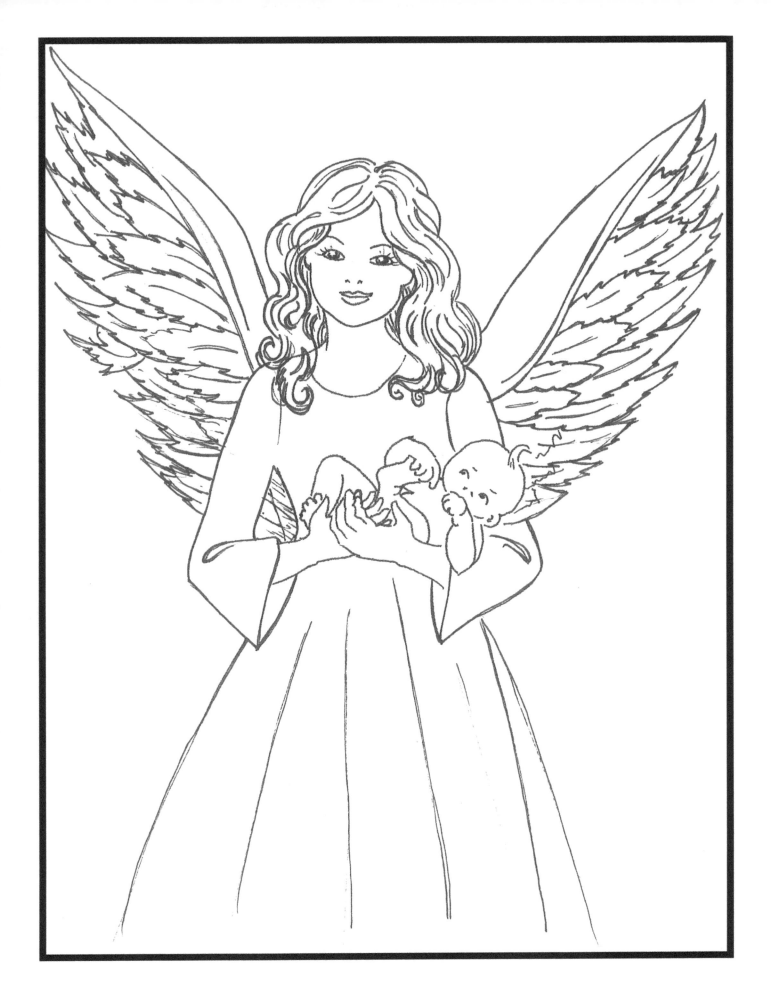

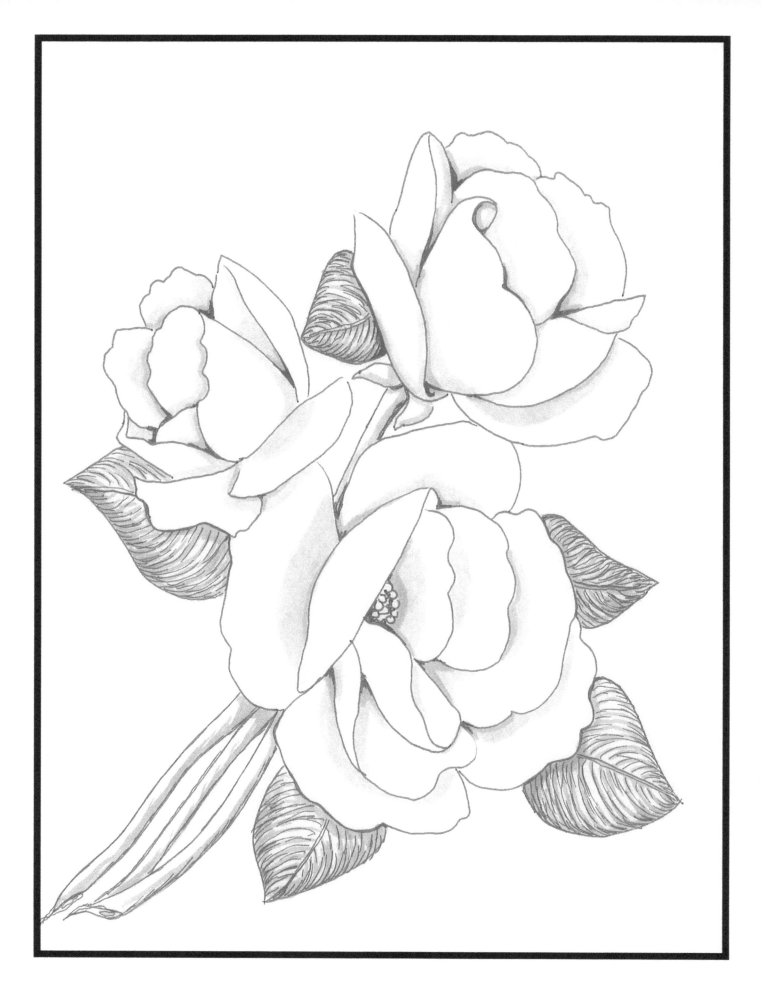

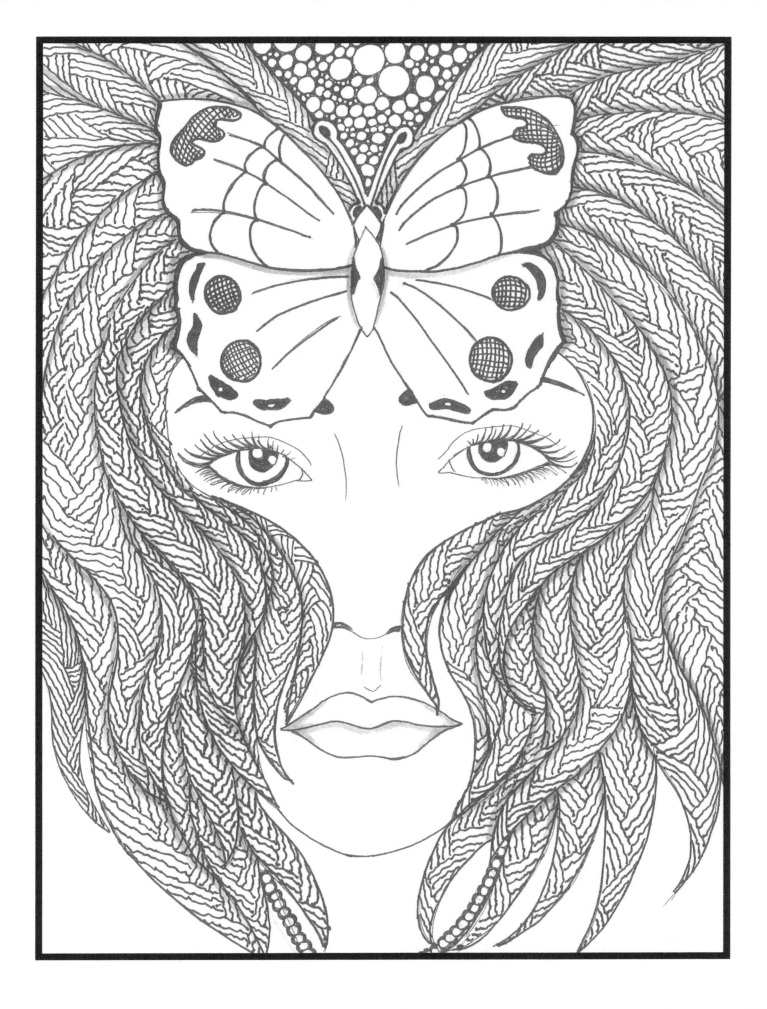

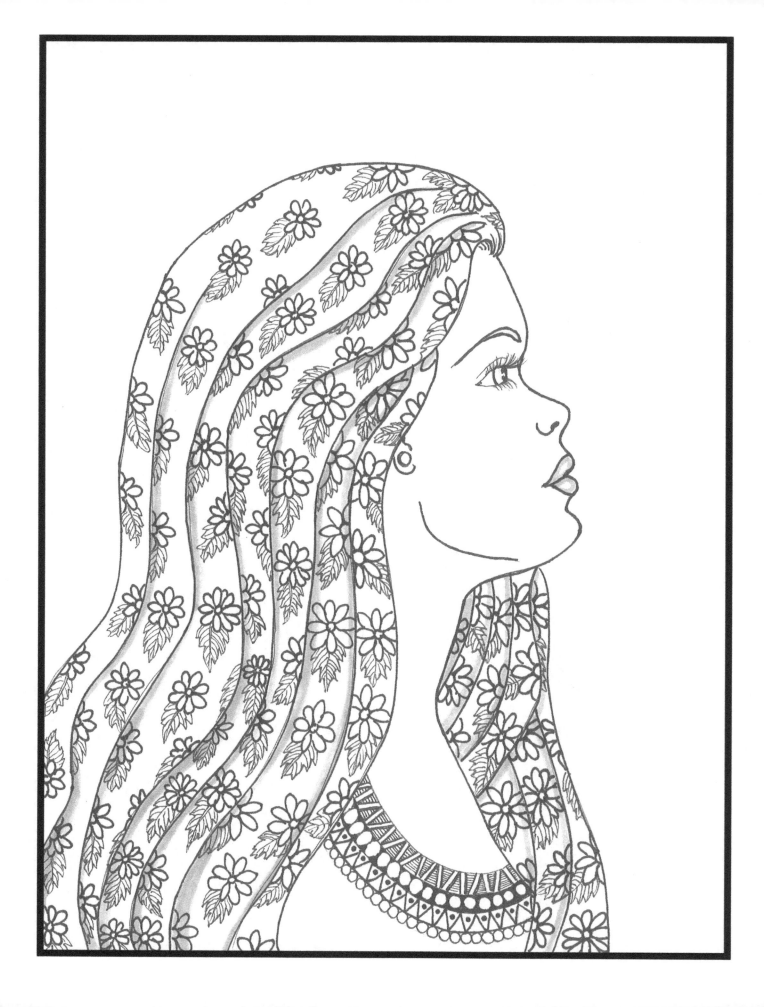

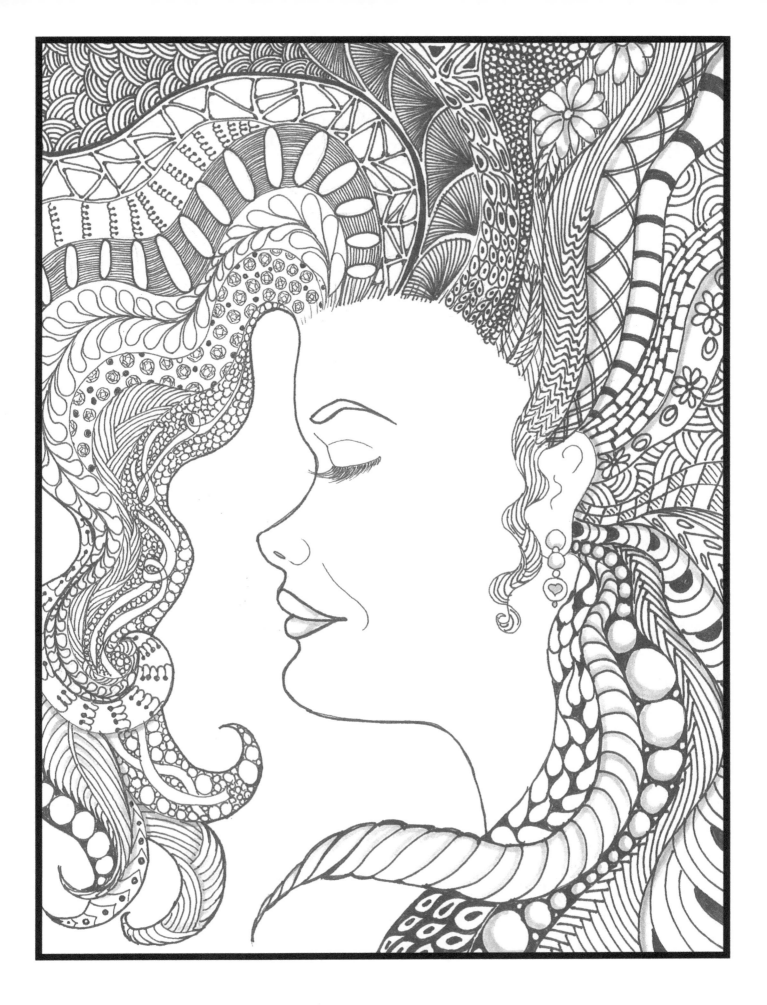

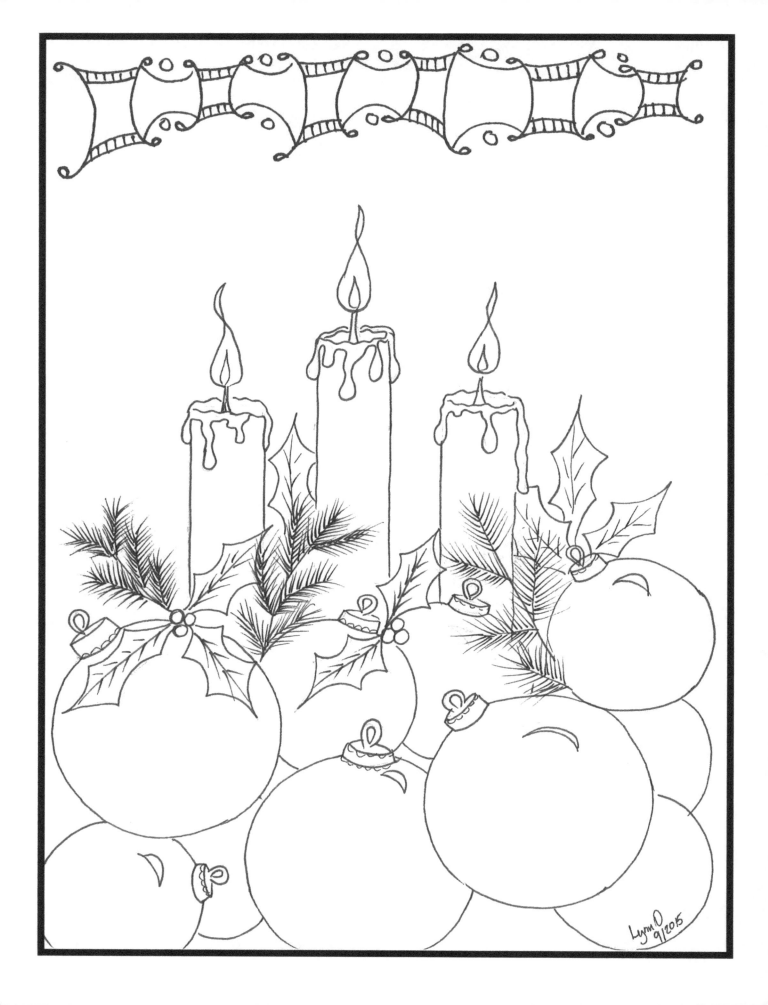

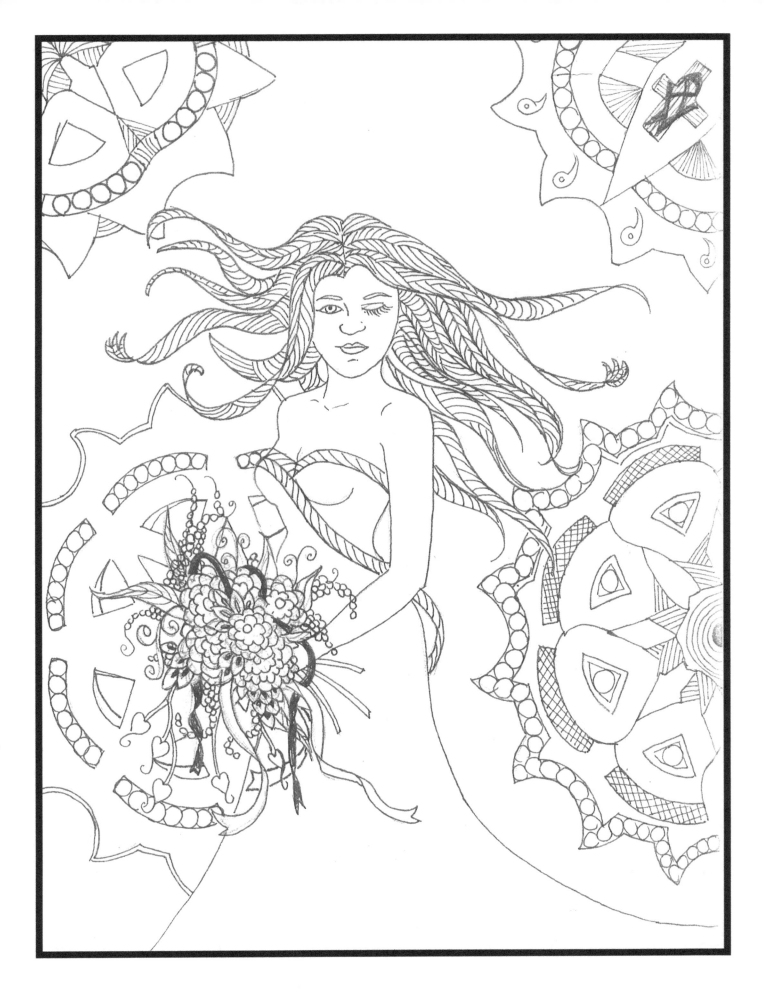

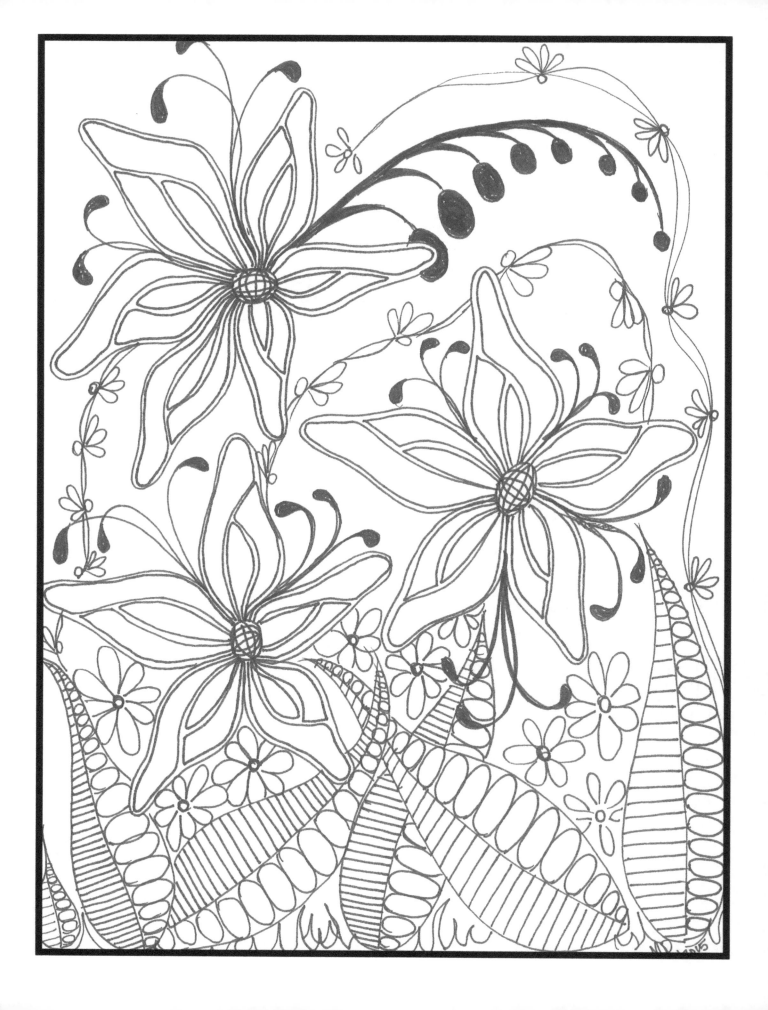

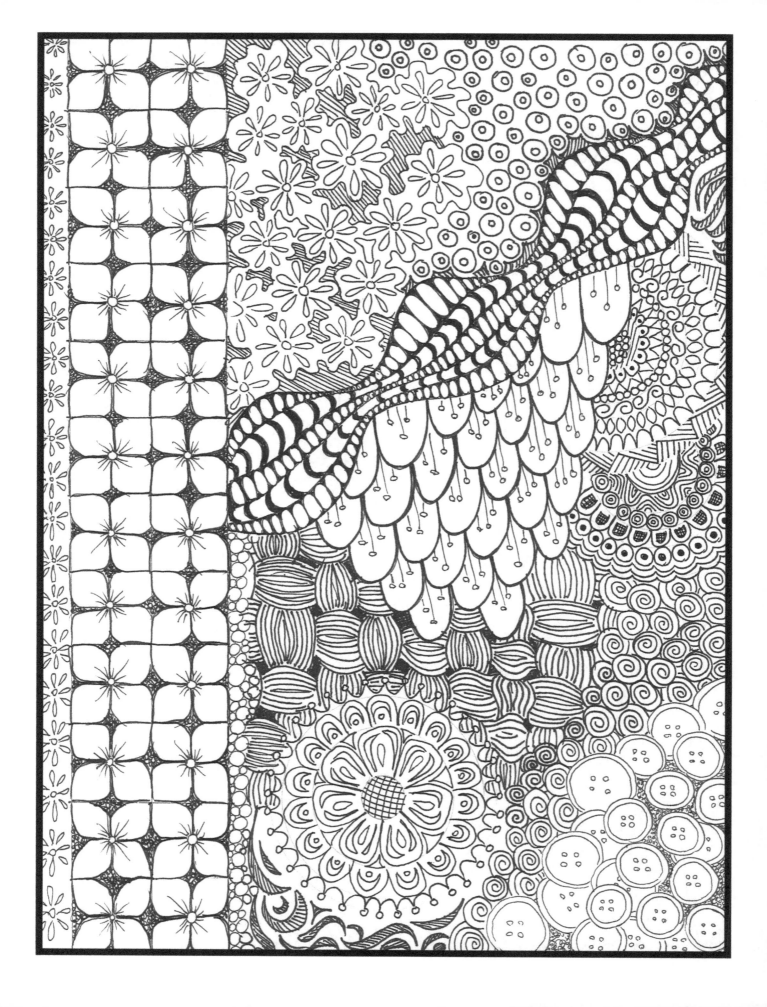

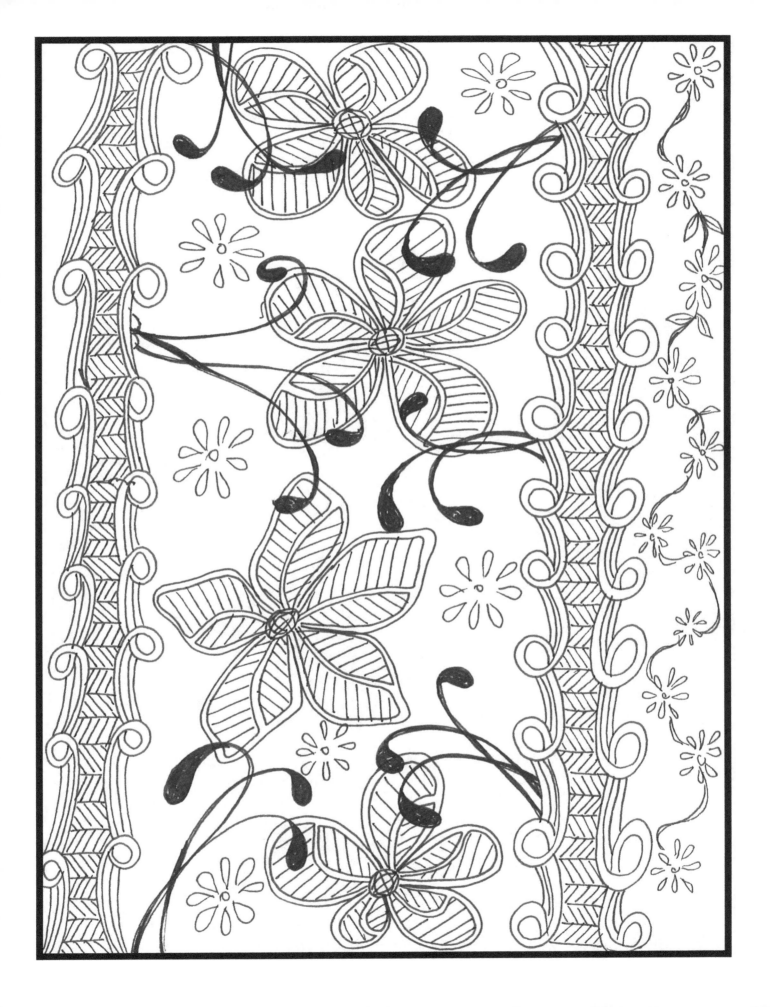

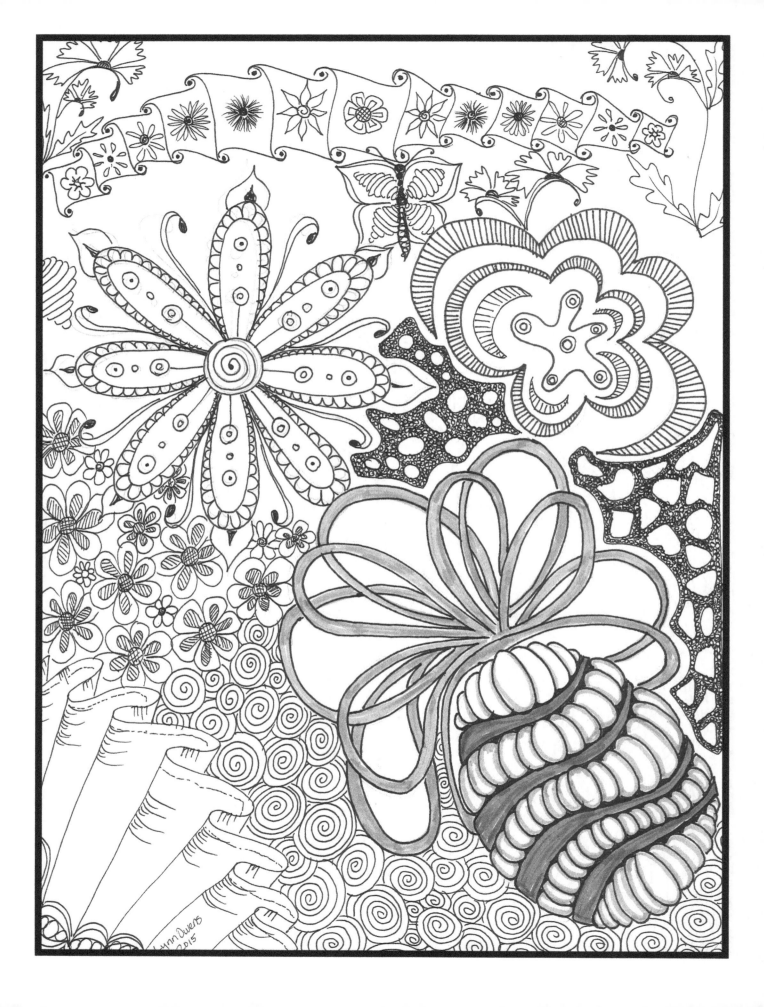

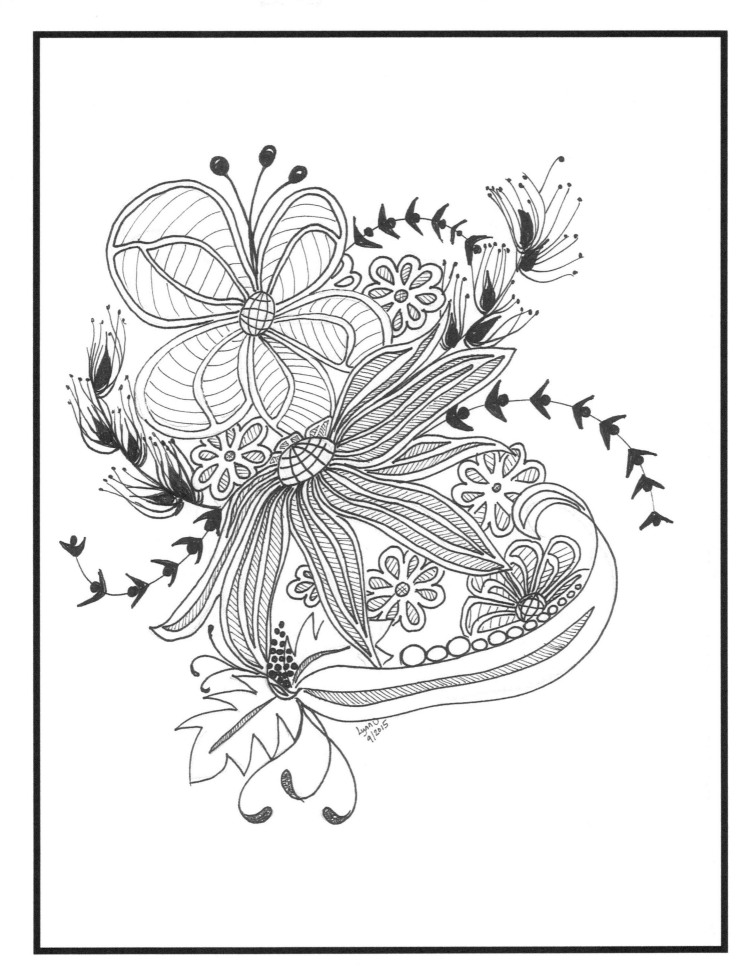

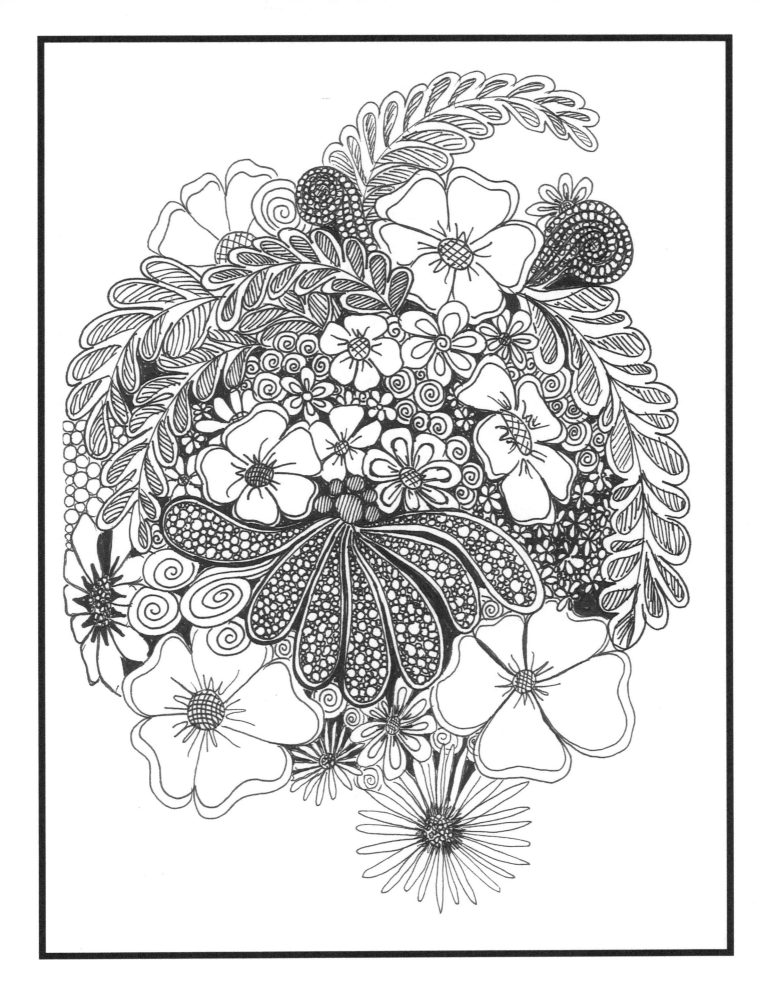

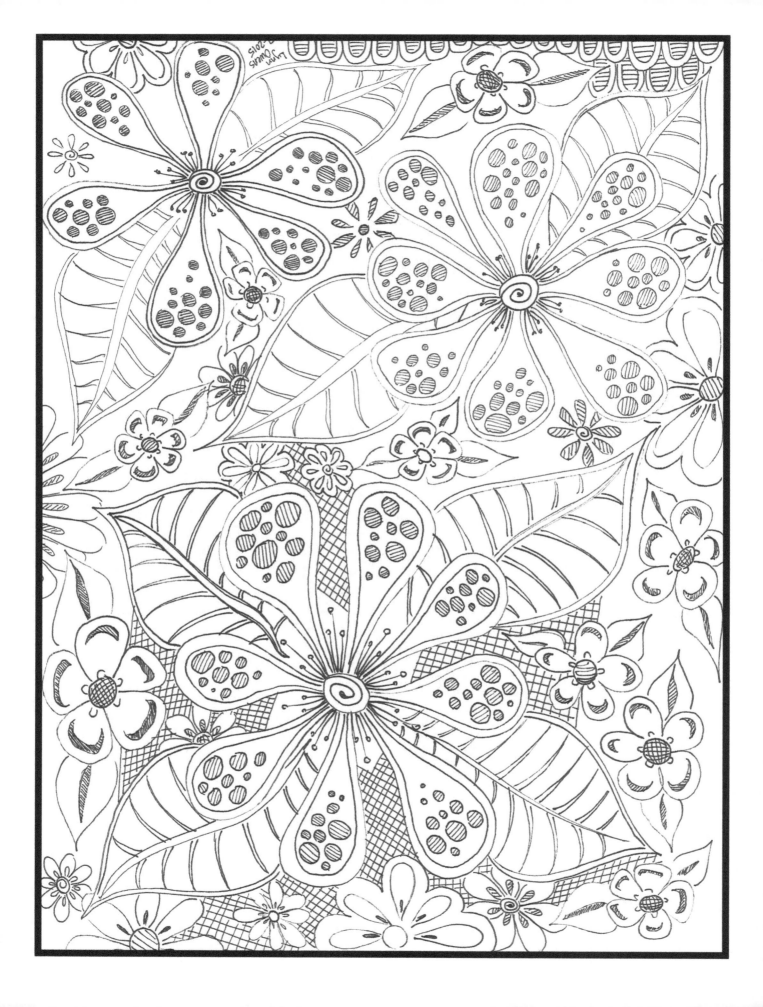

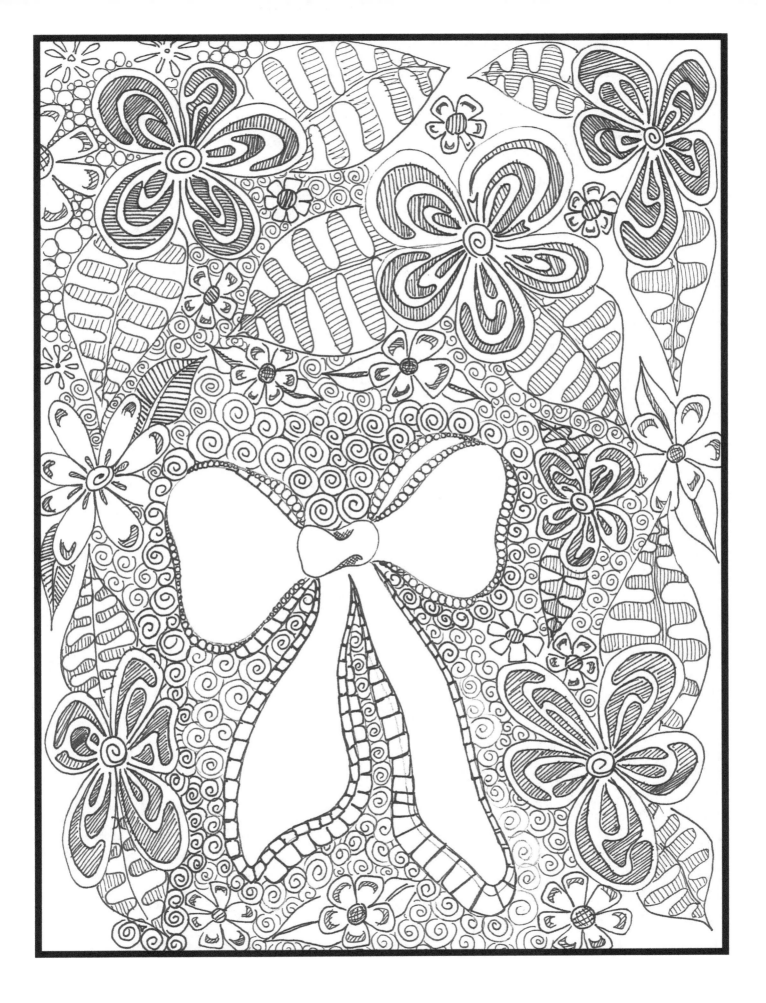

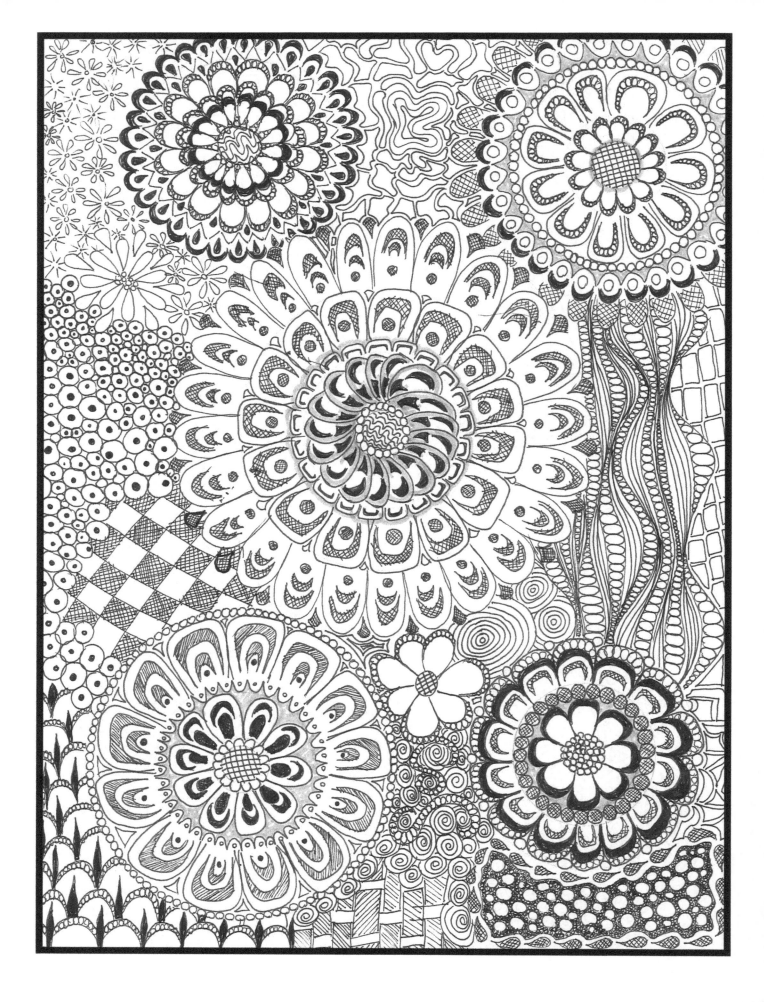

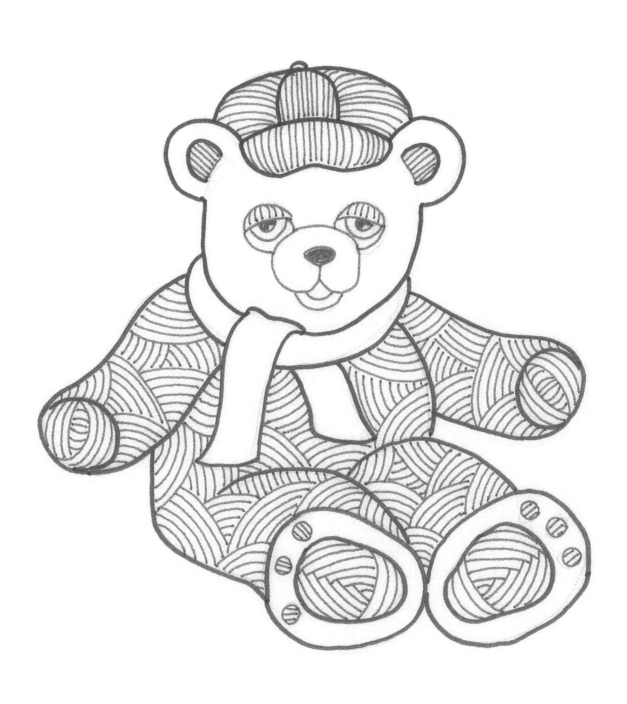

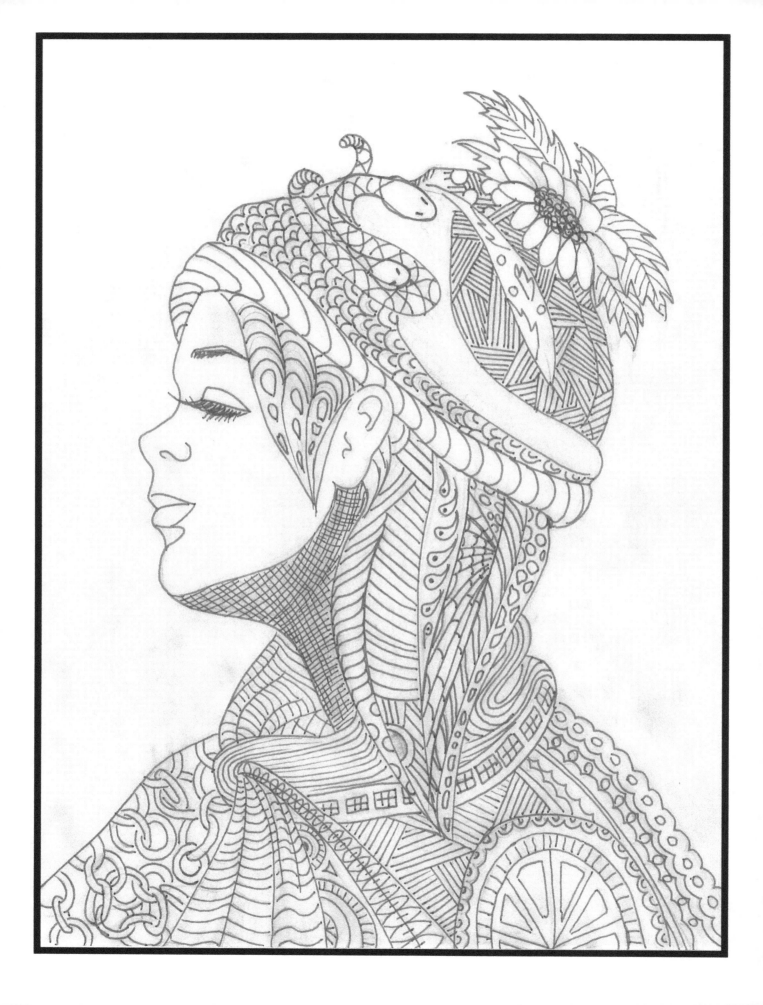

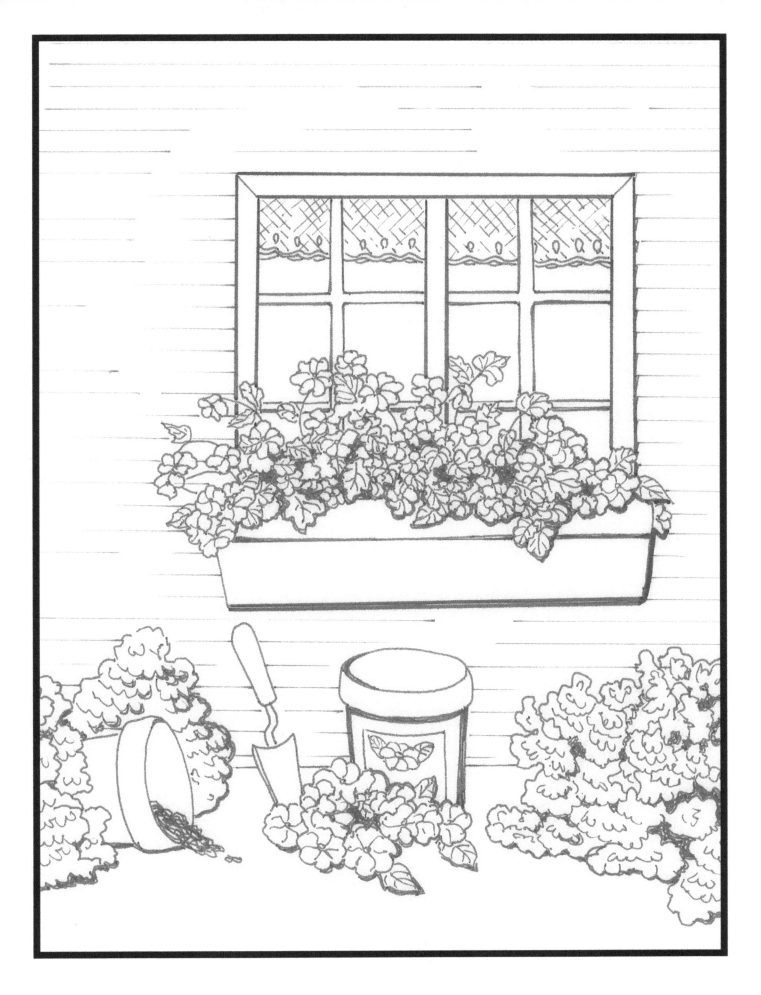

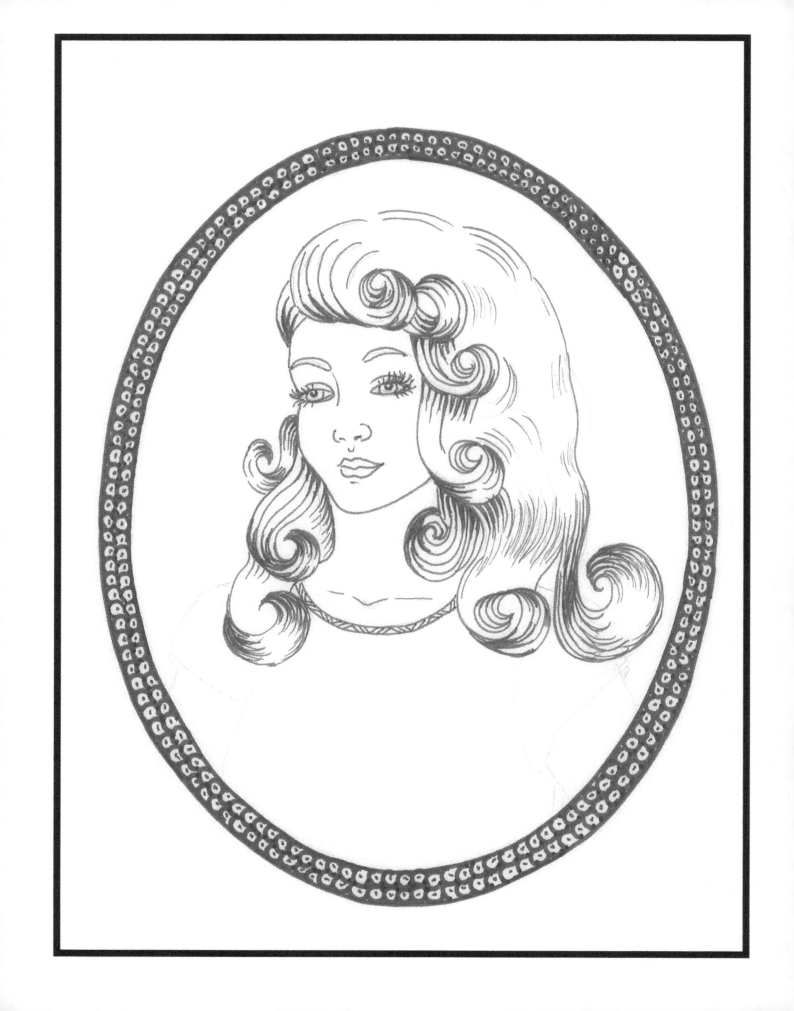

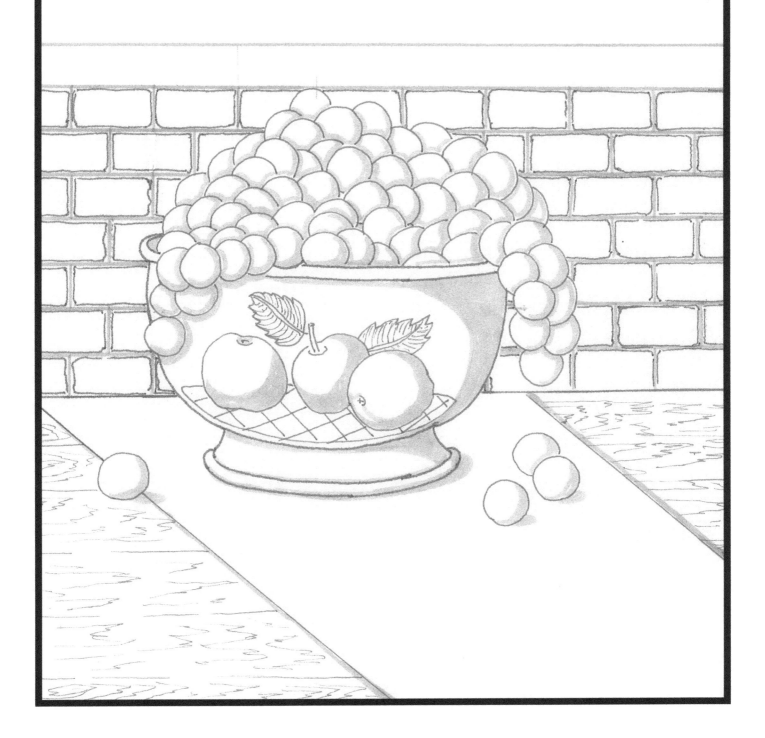

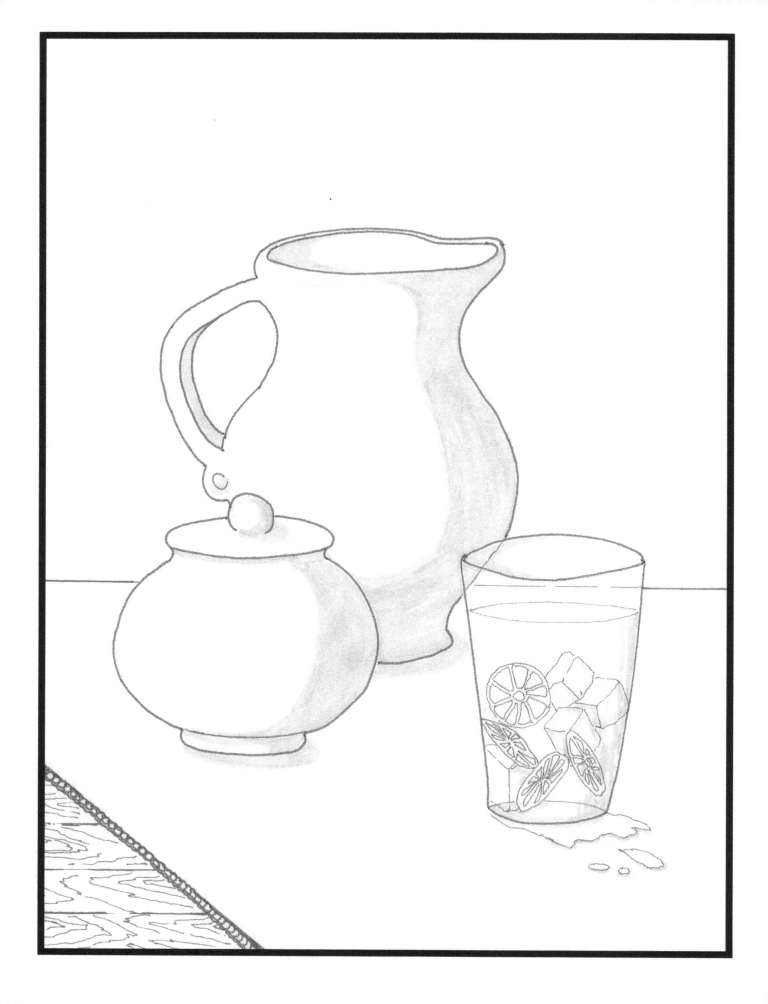

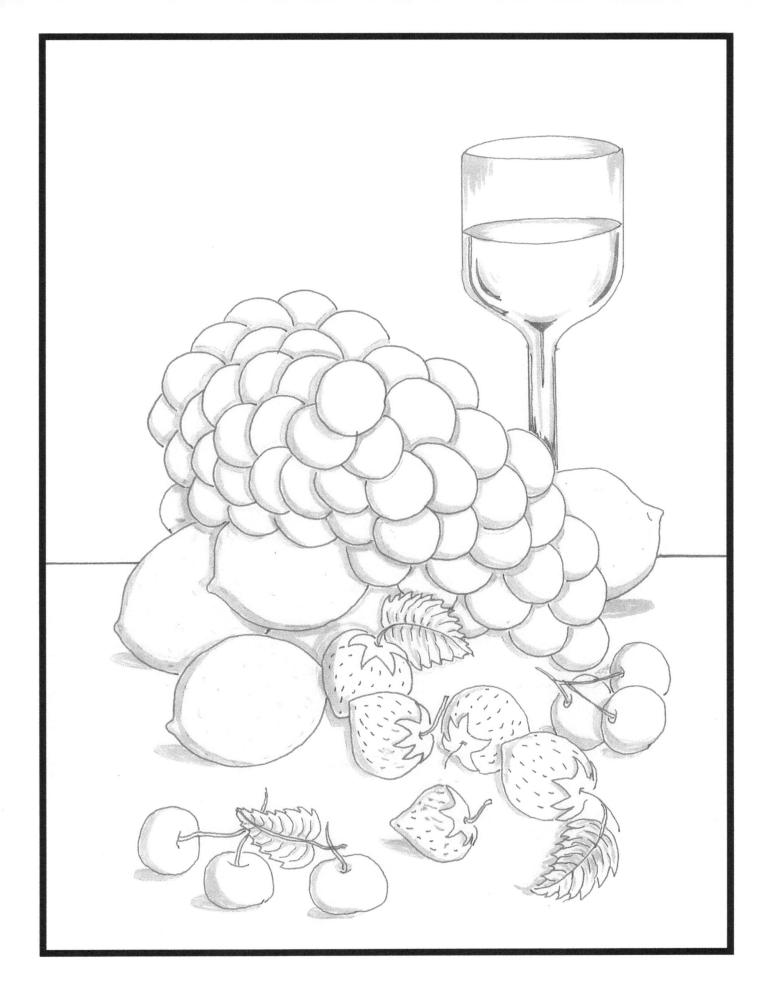

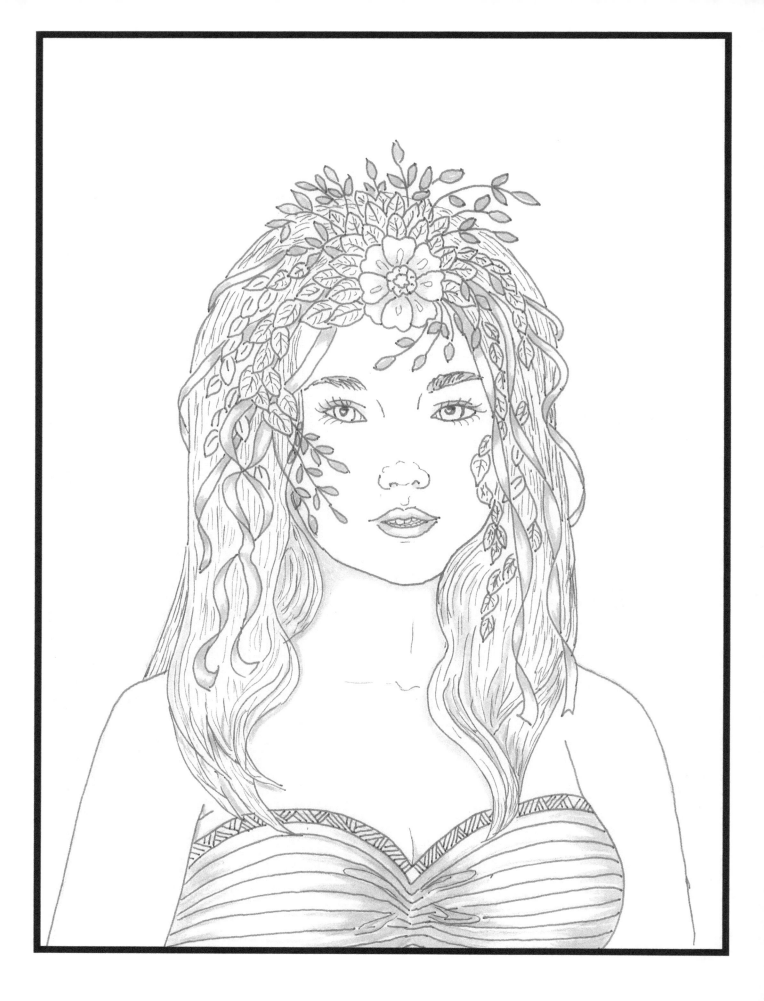

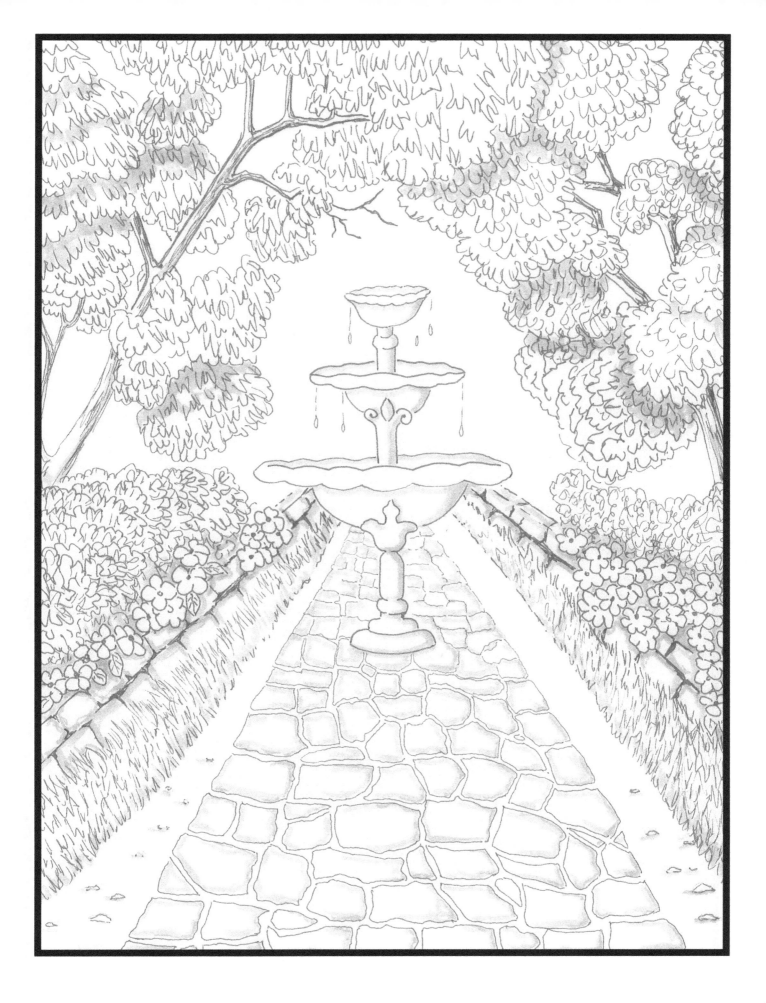

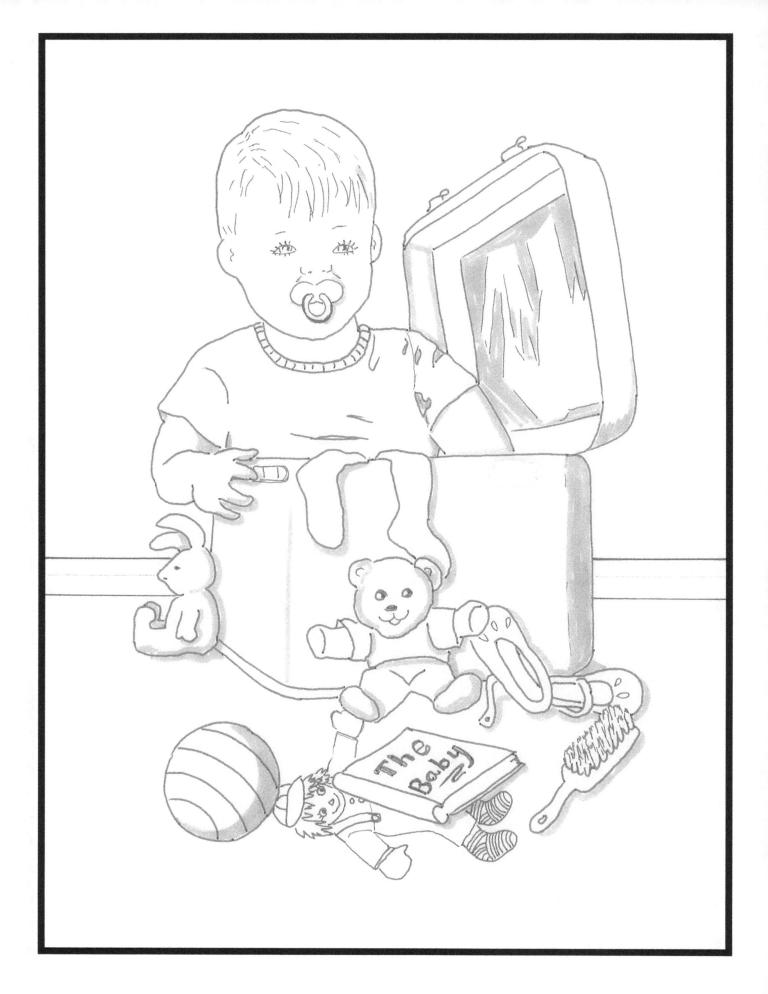

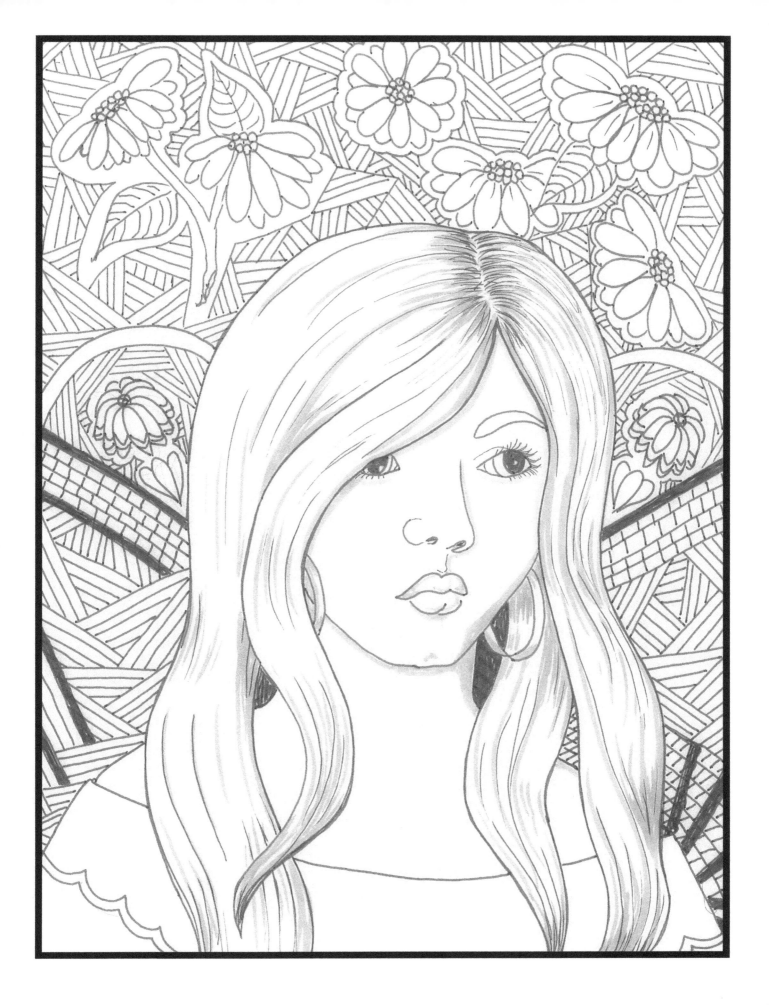

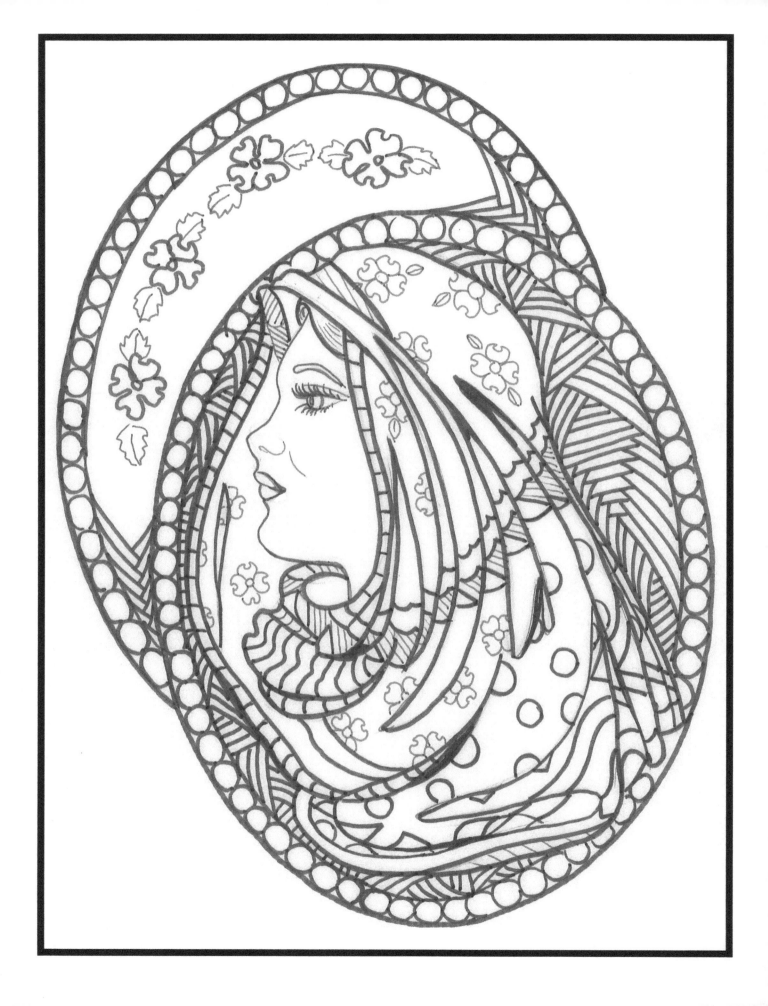

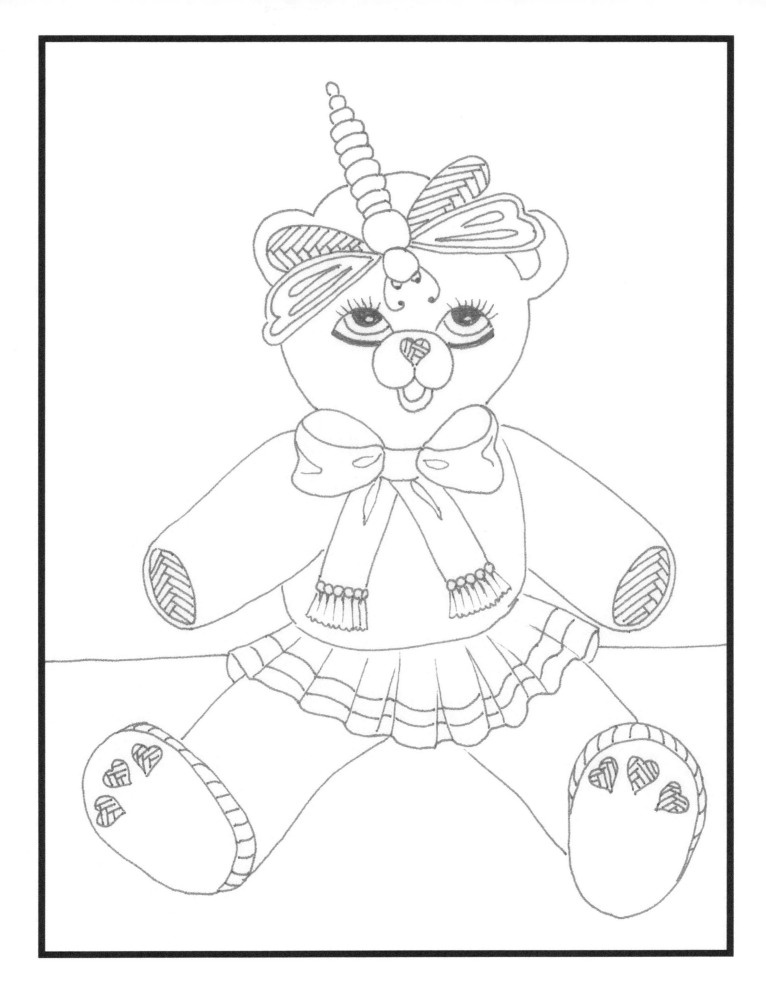

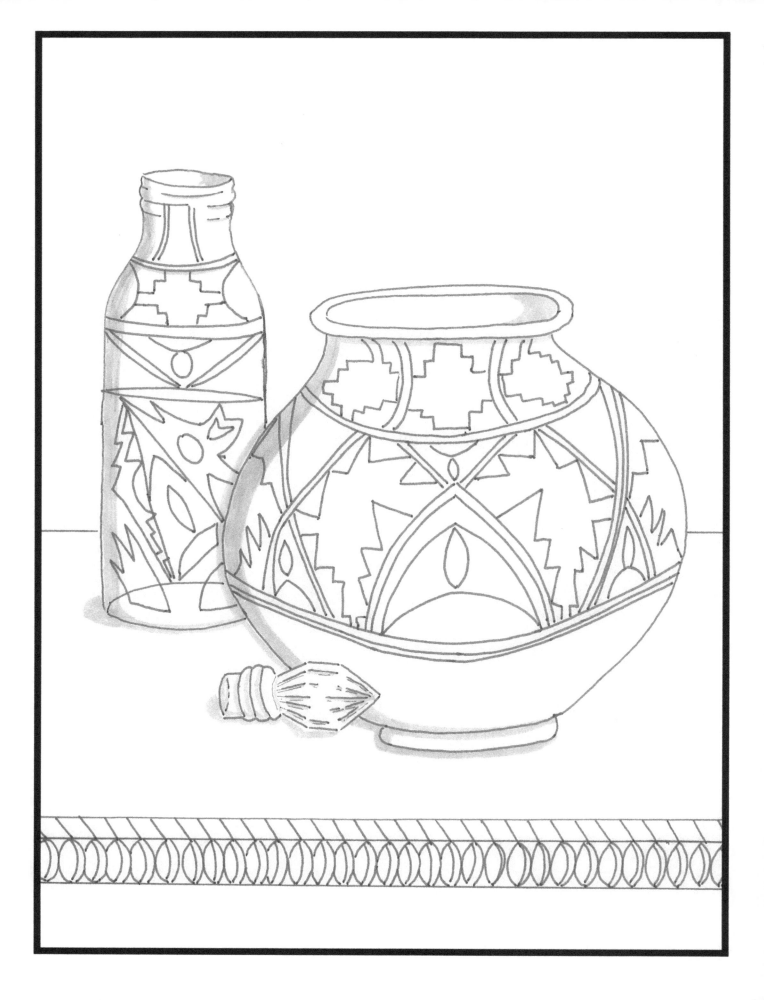

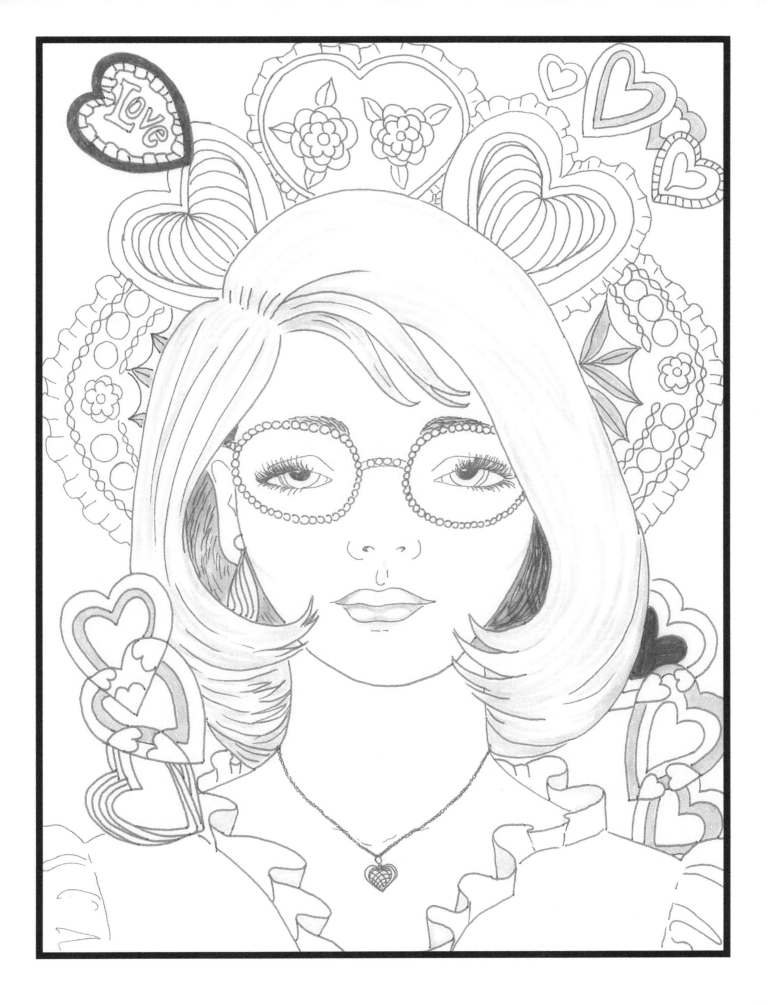

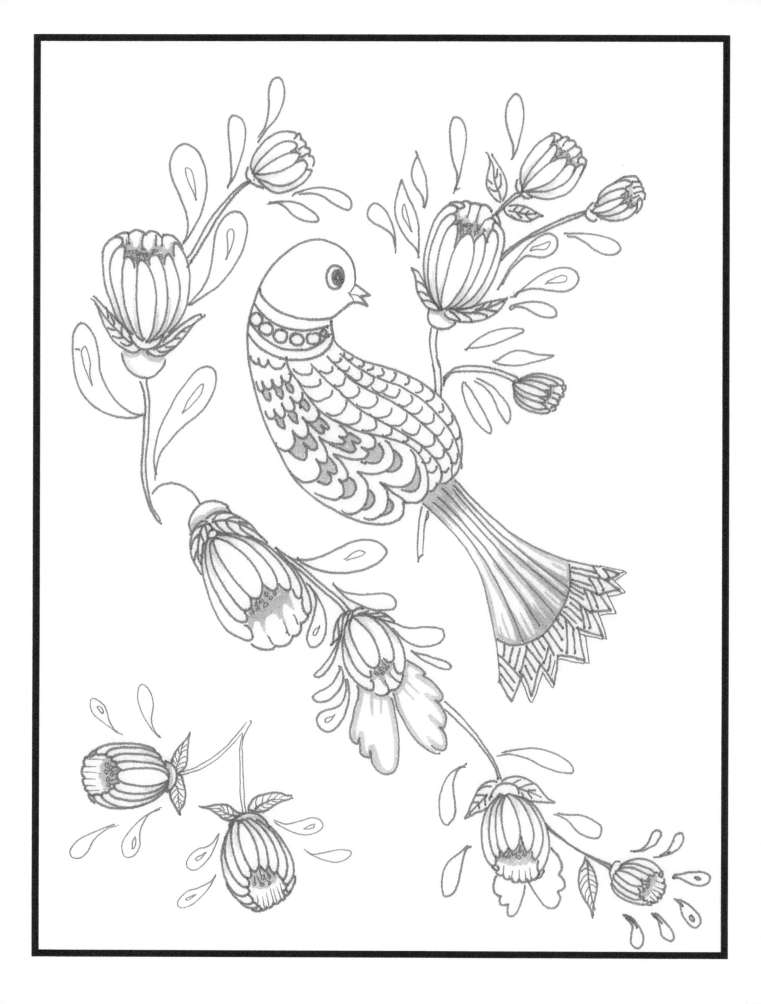

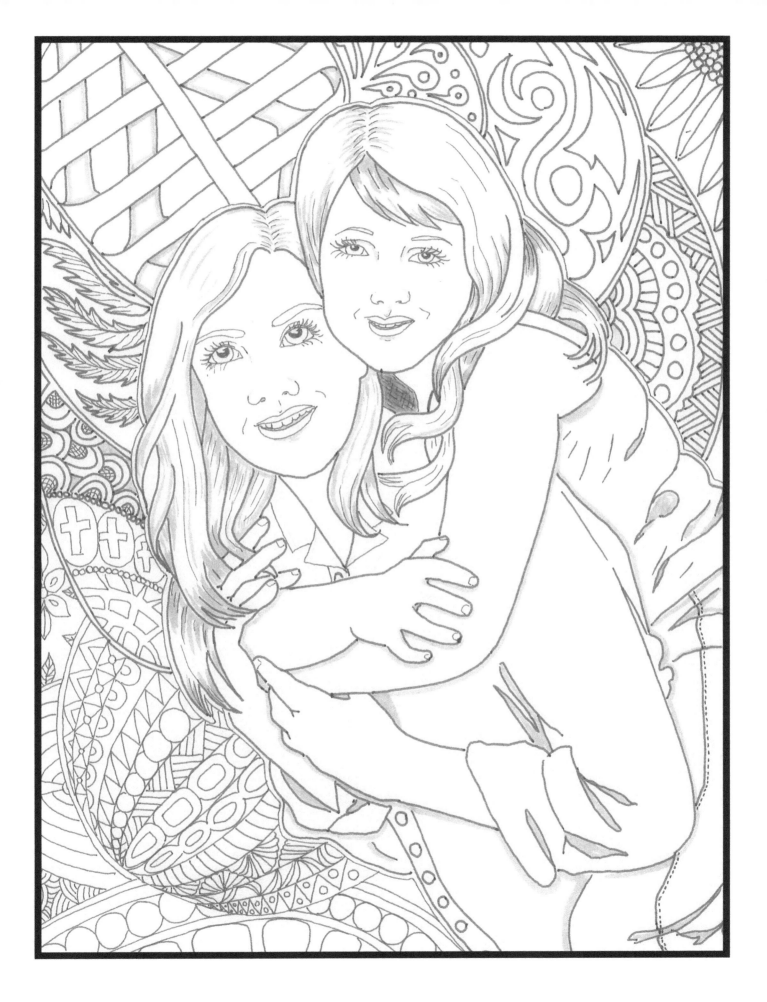

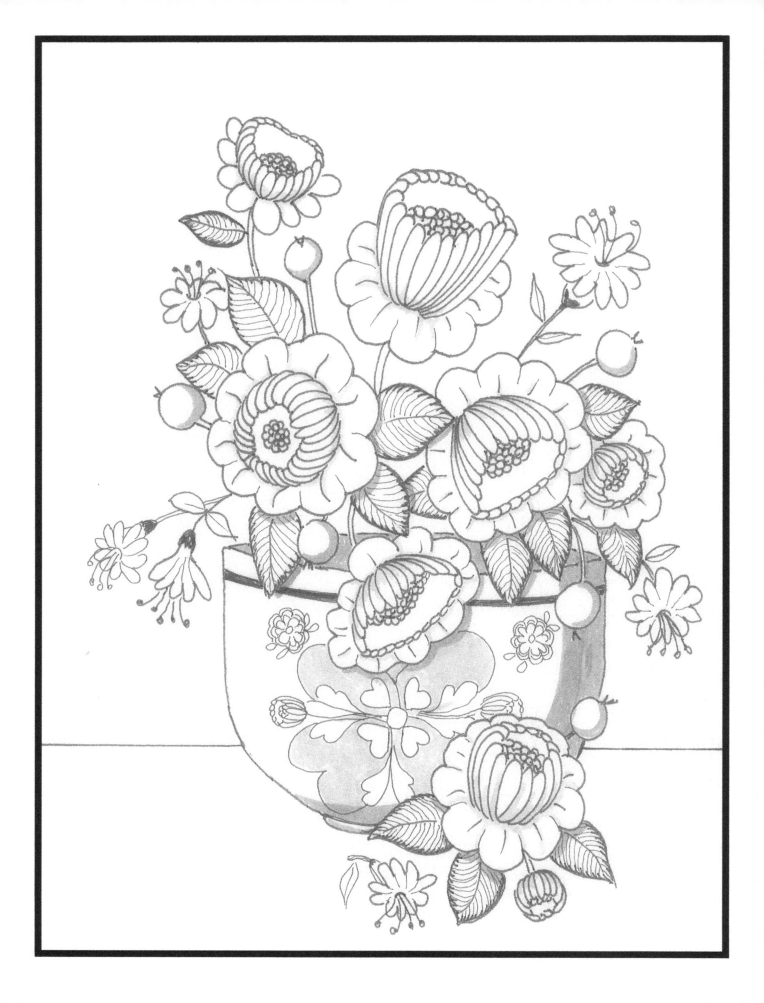

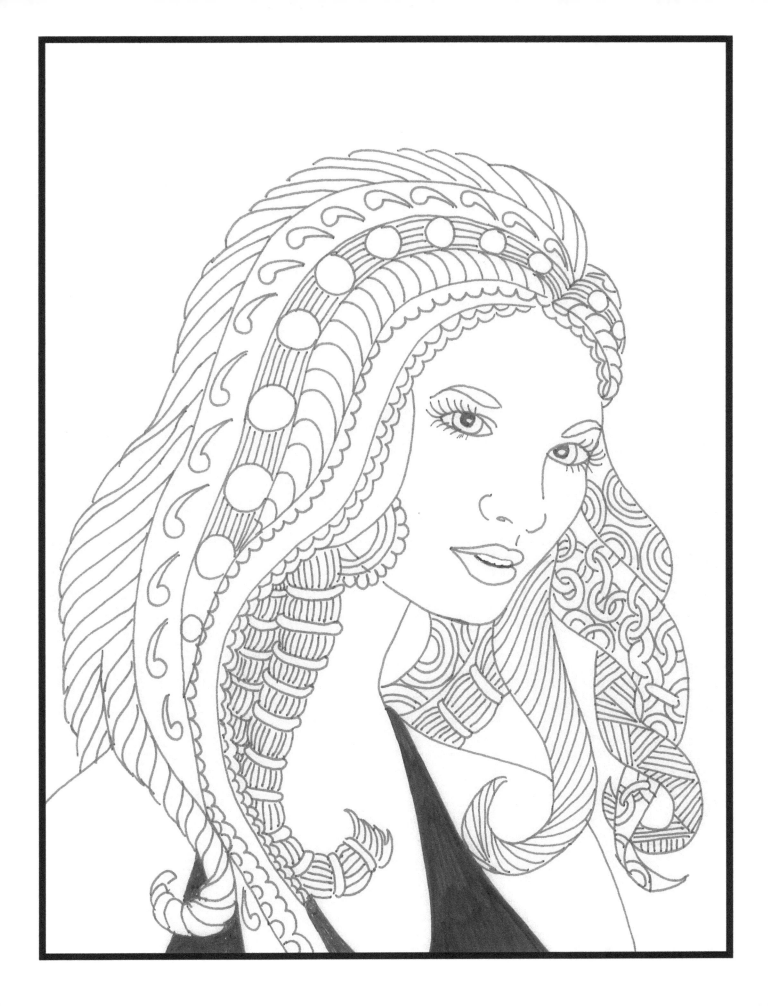

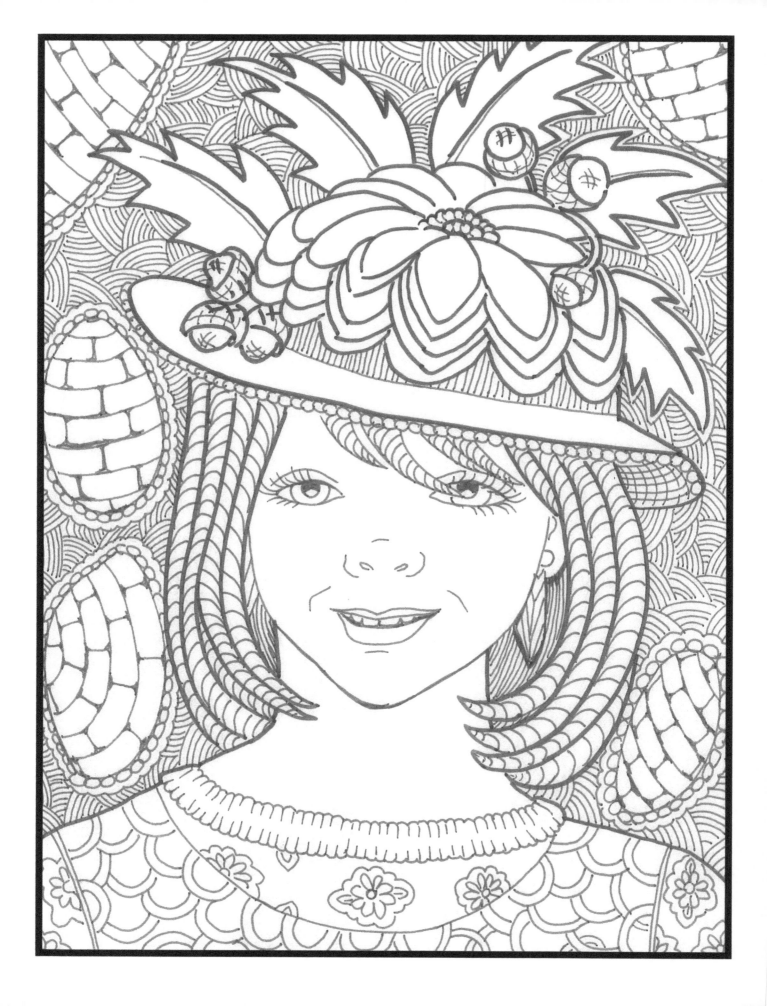

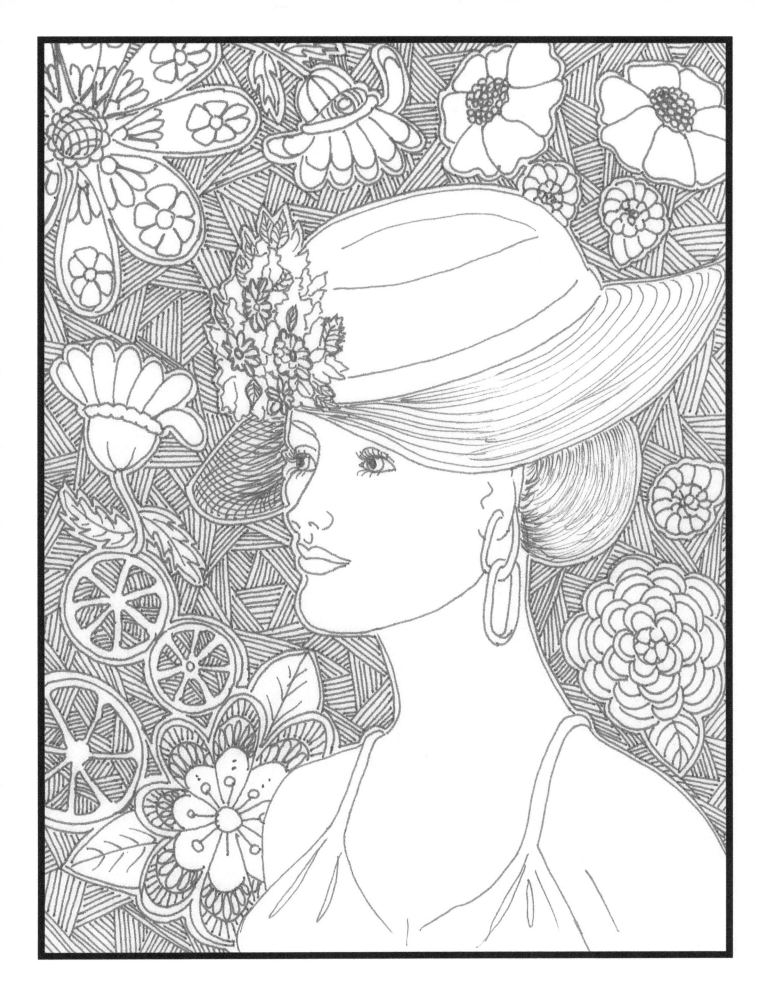

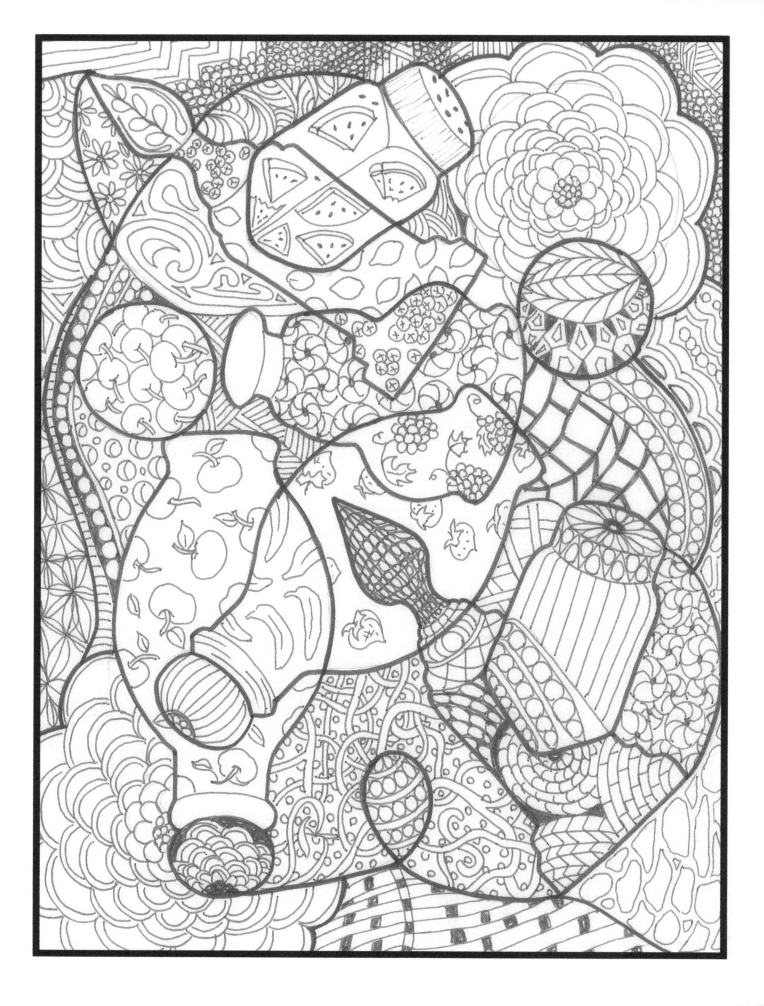

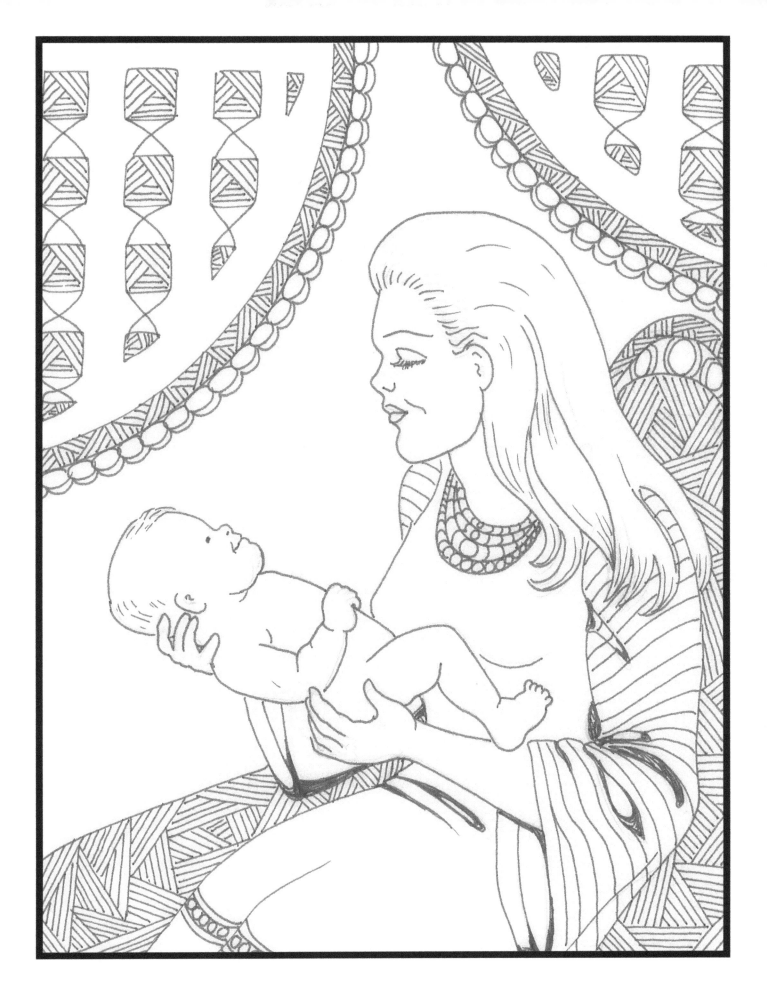

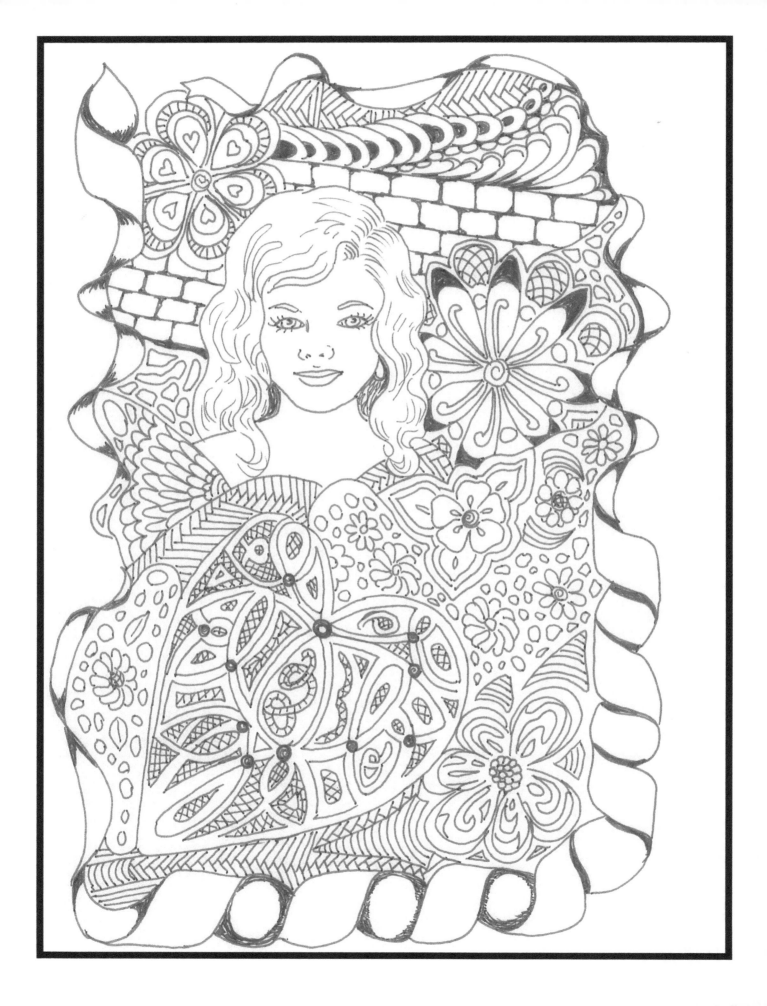

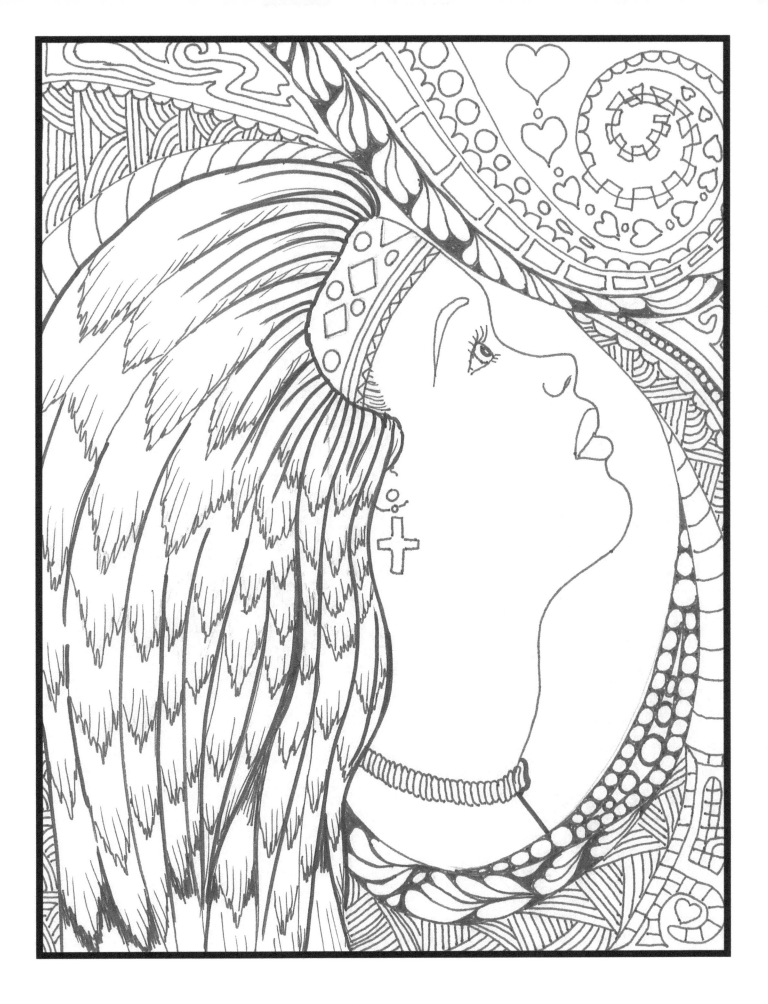

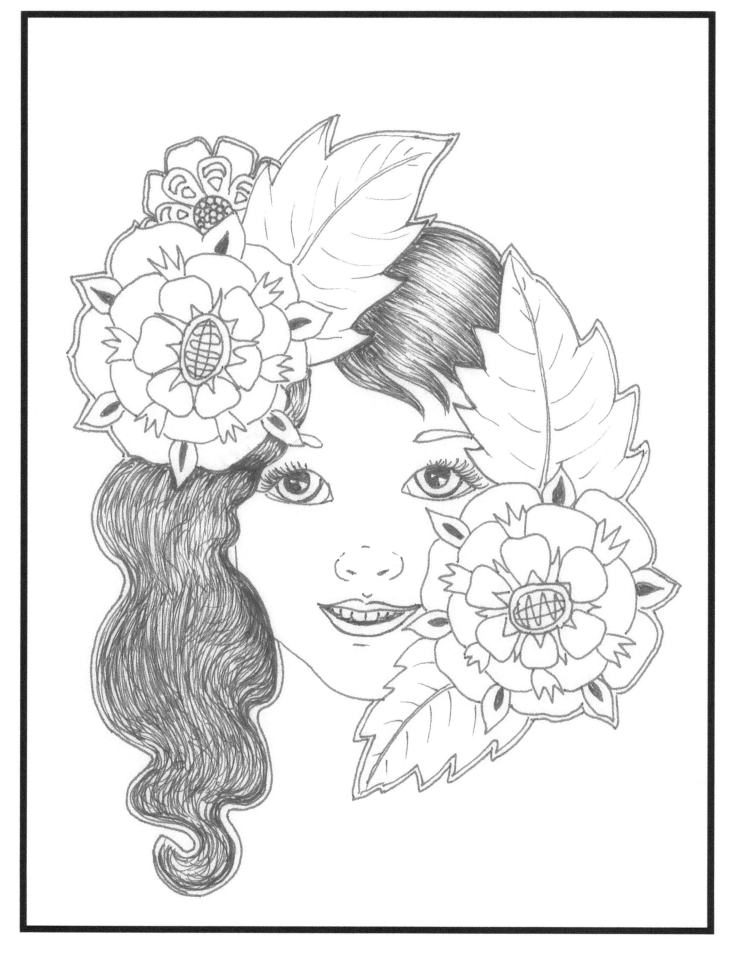

CPSIA information can be obtained
at www.ICGtesting.com
Printed in the USA
LVHW061150151121
703369LV00007B/91

9 781612 254739